The Right Vitamins

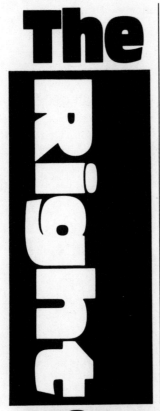

The Right Vitamins

Richard F. Gerson, Ph. D.

Contemporary Books, Inc.
Chicago

Library of Congress Cataloging in Publication Data

Gerson, Richard F.
   The right vitamins.

   Includes index.
   1. Vitamin therapy.   2. Vitamins in human nutrition.
3. Minerals in nutrition.   I. Title.
RM259.G47   1984   615.8'54   84-14966
ISBN 0-8092-5405-0

Published by Contemporary Books, Inc.
180 North Michigan Avenue, Chicago, Illinois 60601
Manufactured in the United States of America
Library of Congress Catalog Card Number: 84-14966
International Standard Book Number: 0-8092-5405-0

Published simultaneously in Canada by Beaverbooks, Ltd.
195 Allstate Parkway, Valleywood Business Park
Markham, Ontario L3R 4T8 Canada

Contents

1 Introduction

An abundance of information about vitamins and minerals is available in books and magazines, on television and radio. Some of these sources tout the necessity of nutritional supplements, others encourage taking megadoses, and still others make exaggerated claims that vitamin and mineral supplements will provide eternal youth and well-being. Thankfully, there are also authorities who provide accurate information regarding these nutrients without claiming any miracle effects.

Vitamins and minerals basically serve as coenzymes to enhance other bodily functions. These functions can be cellular, such as cell growth and reproduction; glandular, such as hormone production; or organic, such as proper heart and lung function. Just as vitamins and minerals can improve a particular body action, a deficiency of either or both of these nutrients can dramatically reduce the functional efficiency of the body. The result is known as a *deficiency symptom*.

Deficiency symptoms occur when the body does not get a sufficient amount of a particular vitamin or mineral. *Proper intake, through pill supplements or food, will not guarantee a cure for the deficiency symptom if it has already occurred, nor will adequate intake always prevent the onset of a symptom. Appropriate vitamin and mineral intake will help the body function more effectively so that deficiency symptoms probably will not occur or the body's restorative powers will improve so the deficiency can be corrected.*

This book is designed to be an easy-access reference guide, not a substitute for traditional medical and health care. You begin by taking the Self-Test in Chapter 2. The test enables you to identify the specific problems or deficiency symptoms you may have, as well as the vitamins and minerals that can remedy the problem. Once you have identified those problems, you proceed to Chapter 3. In this chapter, you will find an alphabetical listing and a description of common health problems and nutritional deficiency symptoms. Additionally, there is information on how an adequate intake of the proper vitamins and minerals can alleviate the problems, and which foods provide those vitamins and minerals.

The next step is to read Chapter 4. Here you will find a listing of each vitamin and mineral that is associated with a given problem. There is also a description of the function of the nutrient, other deficiency symptoms that may be related to it, and the best food sources for the nutrient. This chapter may be used as a cross-reference for the previous chapter.

The final step in using this book is to turn to the appendix, which lists all of the information in the book in chart form. The chart provides daily dosages of each nutrient, based on the Recommended Daily Allowance and supplemental intake ranges. There is also information on food sources and a list of the deficiency symptoms associated with each vitamin and mineral.

The information in this book has been provided with you in mind. It is easily available for repeated reference. It is also my fervent hope that you will develop sound nutritional habits so this book becomes unnecessary.

2 | Self-Test

The following self-test will help you identify certain conditions or symptoms you may have and how they may be alleviated by taking the right vitamin or mineral. Once you have identified the conditions that affect you, turn to Chapter 3 to find out more about them.

If you experience:	Then you need more:
Abdominal cramps	Pantothenic Acid
Acne	B Complex, Zinc
Alcoholism	A, B Complex, C, D, Iron, Magnesium, Potassium, Zinc
Allergies	A

If you experience:	Then you need more:
Anemia	Iron, B_6, B_{12}, Folic Acid, C
Angina pectoris	E, F, Inositol, Niacin
Appetite loss	A, B_1, Niacin, Phosphorus, Sodium
Arthritis	B_6
Asthma	A, B_{12}, F, Manganese
Atherosclerosis	B_6, Chromium
Athlete's foot	A
Backache	C
Baldness	B Complex, C, E, F
Bedsores	B Complex, C
Beriberi	B_1
Bleeding gums	C
Bleeding stomach ulcer	Choline
Blemishes	A
Body odor	B_{12}
Brittle nails	F
Bronchitis	A, C
Bruises	C
Burns	PABA, Zinc
Bursitis	B_6, C, Magnesium
Cancer	A, C
Canker sores	Niacin
Cardiac arrest	B Complex, Calcium, Potassium
Capillary wall ruptures	C
Cataracts	B_2
Colds	C
Constipation	B Complex, Potassium
Convulsions	B_6

If you experience:	Then you need more:
Cystitis	A, C, D, E, B Complex
Dandruff	B_6, B_{12}, F
Dehydration	Sodium
Dental cavities	C, D, Calcium
Depression	B Complex
Dermatitis	B Complex
Diabetes	A, B_1, B_2, E, Chromium, Potassium, Zinc
Diarrhea	D, F, Pantothenic Acid
Digestive disturbances	B Complex, C
Dizziness	B_2, B_6
Drowsiness	Biotin
Dry hair	A, B Complex, E, F, Iodine
Duodenal ulcers	Pantothenic Acid
Eczema	F, Inositol, Pantothenic Acid
Edema	B_6
Emotional instability	B_1
Fatigue	A, B complex, Phosphorus, Zinc
Gallstones	F
Gastritis	B Complex, C
Gingivitis	C
Glucose intolerance	Chromium
Gray hair	Folic Acid, PABA
Growth problems	B_2, Choline, Folic Acid, Zinc
Halitosis	Niacin
Hay fever	B Complex, C
Headaches	Niacin, PABA
Heart palpitations	Calcium
Hemorrhaging	C, K

If you experience:	Then you need more:
Hepatitis	C
High cholesterol	F, Inositol
Hypertension	Choline
Hypoglycemia	Pantothenic Acid
Hypothyroidism	D, Iodine
Hysteria	B_6
Impotence	E
Indigestion	B_1, B_2
Infertility	E, Zinc
Insomnia	B Complex, D, Calcium
Intestinal disorders	Pantothenic Acid
Intestinal gas	Sodium
Irritability	B_1
Itching/burning eyes	A, B_2
Kidney dysfunction	Pantothenic Acid
Kidney stones	B_6, Magnesium
Lesions	B_2
Liver dysfunction.	Choline
Loss of smell	A
Memory lapses	B Complex, Iron
Memory loss	B_1
Ménière's syndrome	Niacin
Menopausal symptoms	D, E
Menstrual cramps	B Complex, Calcium
Mental illness	Niacin
Miscarriage	E, K
Muscle cramps	Calcium, Pantothenic Acid, Potassium
Muscle spasms	D, Calcium, Phosphoris, Potassium, Sodium

If you experience:	Then you need more:
Myopia	D
Nausea	Niacin
Nerve degeneration	B_{12}
Nervousness	B_1, B_{12}, D, Calcium, Magnesium, Niacin, Pangamic Acid, Phosphorus, Potassium
Nervous tension	B Complex, C
Night blindness	A
Nosebleeds	C, K
Numbness	B_1, Calcium
Obesity	Iodine, Phosphorus
Osteomalacia	D, Calcium, Phosphorus
Osteoporosis	D, Calcium
Pellegra	Niacin
Phlebitis	E
Premature aging	Pantothenic Acid
Prickly heat	C
Psoriasis	A, F
Pyorrhea	C, D, Calcium, Phosphorus
Red sore tongue	B_2
Respiratory failure	B Complex, Potassium
Restlessness	Pantothenic Acid
Rheumatism	B_6, C, D, Calcium
Rickets	D
Rough bumpy skin	A
Rough dry skin	A, B Complex, F, Potassium
Schizophrenia	B Complex, C, E
Shingles	B_{12}
Shortness of breath	B_1, B_{15}

If you experience:	Then you need more:
Sinus trouble	A
Skin pallor	Iron
Skin sores	Copper
Soft tooth enamel	A, D, Calcium
Sterility	E, Zinc
Stress	All vitamins & minerals
Sunburn	PABA
Susceptibility to infections	A, C
Tetany	Calcium
Tremors	Magnesium
Varicose veins	F
Vitiligo	PABA
Vomiting	Pantothenic Acid, Sodium
Warts	A
Weakness	B_6, B_{12}, Copper, Niacin, Potassium
Weight loss	Phosphorus, Sodium
Xerophthalmia	A

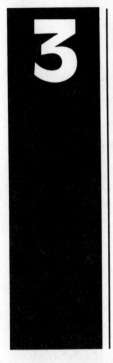

3 | Common Health Problems and Deficiency Symptoms

In this chapter you will find an alphabetical listing of health concerns, some common, some more serious. Some are easily remedied, and others will require the attention of a doctor. In many cases, the problems listed are the result of a deficiency, such as dry skin or a susceptibility to infections. Other problems, such as heart disease or cancer, cannot be cured with vitamins; rather, you can try to prevent the problem from occurring by ingesting certain nutrients. No matter what the problem, you should see a doctor if your condition persists.

Abdominal Cramps

Description: Strong, painful, involuntary contractions of

9

the stomach can be caused by a reaction to food. The problem can also be due to a lack of pantothenic acid, one of the B complex vitamins. Pantothenic acid helps regulate the proper metabolism of carbohydrates, proteins, and fats. The vitamin also aids in the formation of nerve-regulating hormones. The combination of these functions can prevent the stomach from cramping.

Dosage: You need .5–10 mg of pantothenic acid a day.

Food Sources: This vitamin is supplied by brewer's yeast, legumes, organ meats, salmon, wheat germ, whole grains, mushrooms, and orange juice.

Acne

Description: This skin disorder is characterized by an inflammation of the oil glands and hair follicles of the body. The disease is most evident in the facial area, but other parts of the body may be affected as well. The disorder is characterized by blackheads and pus pimples. Adolescents and teenagers are most likely to be affected, and the condition can clear up as adulthood approaches. However, severe acne can leave scars that remain evident for life.

Acne is related to deficiencies in the vitamin B complex, vitamin F, potassium, and zinc. When proper levels of these nutrients are present, acne can be cleared up or prevented in some cases. The B complex vitamins facilitate metabolism and energy production, which lead to proper cell function. Vitamin F promotes glandular activity and removes unnecessary oils and fats from the system. Potassium aids in cell growth and nervous system function. Finally, zinc serves a regulatory function for metabolic processes as well as making more vitamin A available for healthy cell development. It is the combination of these nutrients, with their major contributions being to promote cell growth and metabolism, that has a healing effect on acne.

Dosage: There is no single recommended dosage for the B complex vitamins. There are so many of them that each one is recommended in a variable amount. The RDAs for vitamins are listed on the chart in the appendix. There is no specific daily requirement for vitamin F, except that at least 10 percent of your total calories should be consumed as unsaturated fatty acids. You should have 100–300 mg of potassium every day, and about 15–25 mg of zinc.

Food Sources: Vitamin B complex can be found in brewer's yeast, blackstrap molasses, wheat germ, whole grains, and organ meats. Vitamin F is found in vegetable oils, wheat germ, and sunflower seeds. Potassium comes from dates, figs, peaches, tomato juice, bananas, baked potatoes, raisins, blackstrap molasses, and sunflower seeds. Zinc is found in brewer's yeast, liver, seafood, sunflower seeds, soybeans, spinach, and mushrooms.

Obviously, many of these nutrients come from the same foods, and that is why their combination can be so effective in healing acne.

Alcoholism

Description: This is not so much a symptom as it is a disease. Mild alcoholism, or intoxication, is associated with some loss of muscular coordination and an impairment of mental processes. These effects disappear as the alcohol passes through the system. Chronic alcoholism is the compulsive use of alcohol, and it is considered the disease state. Alcoholism may be a psychiatric disorder, the result of a metabolic defect, or a means of escape from the pressures of life. An alcoholic is physically addicted and then becomes psychologically addicted.

Although vitamin deficiencies have never been implicated as a cause of alcoholism, vitamin therapy is often used during the treatment process. The vitamins that are used most often are A, B complex, C, and D; minerals commonly used are iron, magnesium, potassium, and zinc. These nutrients aid in cell growth, metabolism, nervous system function, and red blood cell production. These functions help the body resist the effects of alcohol and eventually decrease the addictive dependency.

Dosage: You need 5,000 IU of vitamin A daily. The B complex vitamins have individual dosages that are given in the chart in the appendix. You should also get 60 mg of vitamin C, 400 IU of vitamin D, 10–18 mg of iron, 300–350 mg of magnesium, no specific dosage of potassium (but 300–500 mg is suggested), and 15 mg of zinc a day.

Food Sources: Vitamin A comes from green and yellow fruits and vegetables (apricots, spinach, raw carrots, etc.), milk, fish liver oil, and beef liver. The basic sources of the vitamin B complex are blackstrap molasses, brewer's yeast, liver, wheat germ, and whole grains. Vitamin C is found in citrus fruits, cantaloupe, green peppers, broccoli, and potatoes. You get vitamin D from egg yolks, organ meats, bone meal, sunlight, beef liver, milk, salmon, and tuna fish. Iron is supplied by blackstrap molasses, eggs, fish, organ meats, poultry, and wheat germ. Magnesium is found in bran, honey, green vegetables, nuts, seafood, spinach, bone meal, kelp tablets, and tuna fish. You receive potassium from dates, figs, peaches, tomato juice, blackstrap molasses, peanuts, raisins, seafood, apricots, bananas, potatoes, and green peppers. Finally, you get zinc from brewer's yeast, liver, seafood, soybeans, spinach, sunflower seeds, and mushrooms.

Allergies

Description: An allergy is a sensitivity to a substance that does not normally cause a reaction. Examples of allergens include pollens (hay fever), foods, bee stings, and climate changes. It is often thought that allergies are caused by a protein deficiency, but many allergies are caused by insufficient intake of vitamins A and F.

Vitamin A helps you prevent allergic reactions by promoting tissue repair (new and strong cells) and building a resistance to infection. Vitamin F contributes by promoting glandular activity, cell growth, and vital organ respiration. The combination of these vitamins enables the body's cells to function in an appropriate manner, thereby reducing the possibility of an abnormal (allergic) reaction.

Dosage: You should have a minimum of 5,000 IU of vitamin A daily, while vitamin F should constitute approximately 10 percent of your total caloric consumption.

Food Sources: Vitamin A is found in green and yellow fruits and vegetables (especially carrots), milk, and fish liver oil. Vitamin F comes from vegetable oils, wheat germ, and sunflower seeds.

Anemia

Description: Anemia involves a reduction in the number of circulating red blood cells. Many people often refer to anemia as "iron-poor blood" or "tired blood." This is because not enough oxygen is getting to the various cells due to the decreased circulation of red blood cells. However, iron is not the only nutrient that is lacking in an anemic person. Vitamins B_6, B_{12}, and folic acid are also insufficiently supplied.

Iron helps combat anemia by aiding the body in cell growth and reproduction and red blood cell formation. The same is true for B_6, B_{12}, and folic acid. Vitamin C seems to protect the other nutrients so they can function properly.

Dosage: It is recommended that adults receive 18–20 mg of iron daily. This may seem a little high, but you must remember that 1–2 mg of iron is lost to the system because of improper absorption. The slightly higher dosage will compensate for that loss.

The other vitamins should be supplied in these amounts: 1.5–1.8 mg of B_6, 3 mcg of B_{12}, 400 mcg of folic acid, and 60 mg of C.

Food Sources: Iron-rich food sources include liver and other organ meats; shellfish; fruits; nuts; spinach and other green, leafy vegetables; whole grains; and blackstrap molasses.

B_6 is found in many of the same foods as iron and in whole grains, brewer's yeast, and brown rice. B_{12} can be found in cheese, fish, milk, cottage cheese, and eggs. Folic acid is plentiful in all the food sources mentioned above. Finally, vitamin C occurs in citrus fruits, cantaloupe, green peppers, broccoli, and potatoes.

Angina Pectoris (Chest Pains)

Description: This is a cardiovascular condition characterized by an insufficient supply of blood and oxygen to the heart and pains in the chest. It is caused by a narrowing of the coronary arteries that may be caused by various factors. Angina pectoris is not necessarily a nutritional deficiency disease, but an adequate intake of appropriate nutrients may help alleviate the problem. These nutrients include inositol, niacin, vitamin E, and vitamin F. All these vitamins are involved in reducing cholesterol levels in the blood, thus preventing hardening of the arteries, which leads to angina pectoris.

Dosage: You need 13–18 mg of niacin and 12–15 IU of vitamin E. There is no specific recommendation for inositol.

Vitamin F should make up 10 percent of your daily caloric intake.

Food Sources: Inositol is found in blackstrap molasses, citrus fruits, brewer's yeast, meat, milk, nuts, vegetables, whole grains, and lecithin. Niacin comes from brewer's yeast, seafood, lean meats, milk, poultry, dessicated liver, and peanuts. Good sources of vitamin E include dark green vegetables, eggs, liver, wheat germ, vegetable oils, oatmeal, and potatoes. Vitamin F occurs in vegetable oils, wheat germ, and sunflower seeds.

Appetite Loss

Description: There are times when people just do not feel like eating. Often, this is due to external, emotional pressures, but it can also be the result of an insufficient supply of certain nutrients. These include vitamins A, B_1, and niacin and the minerals phosphorus and sodium.

All these nutrients promote cellular function in some manner, which will stimulate the appetite because cells need to be nourished to perform. Specifically, vitamin A is involved in tissue repair. This requires energy, which can be supplied only through food. B_1 and niacin both stimulate the appetite and metabolism, as well as produce energy and promote cellular growth. All these functions require nourishment. Phosphorus is also involved in metabolism and energy production. Finally, sodium helps the cells maintain their proper fluid levels so they can function effectively.

Dosage: You should have 5,000 IU of vitamin A daily, 1-1.5 mg of B_1, 13-18 mg of niacin, 800 mg of phosphorus, and no more than 2 g of sodium (a much lower level—300 mg—has been recommended to prevent fluid retention).

Food Sources: Vitamin A is found in green and yellow leafy vegetables, milk, fish liver oil, and carrots. Vitamin B_1 comes from blackstrap molasses, brewer's yeast, brown rice, fish, meat, nuts, poultry, wheat germ, and sunflower seeds, as does niacin. Phosphorus occurs in eggs, fish, grains, meat, poultry, yellow cheese, and yogurt. Sodium is found in salt, in most canned foods, and in cured meats, such as bacon.

Arthritis

Description: Arthritis is an inflammation of a joint that is usually accompanied by pain. In certain instances there may also be a change in the structure of the joint due to its inability to function properly. Many "remedies" have been recommended for arthritis, including aspirin, pain killers, and salves. However, arthritic pain will be controlled best by vitamin B_6. B_6 serves to improve nerve function, and this can lead to a decrease in the inflammation of the joint due to increased mobility of the surrounding musculature.

Dosage: Vitamin B_6 should be taken in small quantities, approximately 1.8 mg per day. Larger doses will be excreted.

Food Sources: B_6 can be found in the foods that contain other B complex vitamins. These foods include blackstrap molasses, brewer's yeast, green leafy vegetables, meat, wheat germ, whole grains, and brown rice.

Asthma

Description: Asthma is a respiratory problem characterized by difficult or labored breathing. Usually, there is also a wheezing or whistling sound, especially when exhaling. Asthma occurs when the muscles of the small air passageways in the lungs go into spasm. This causes the passageways to narrow. There is a concomitant outpouring of mucus, and both these occurrences make breathing more diffucult.

Asthma is thought to be caused by an allergy, but the condition also occurs during times of emotional stress or nutritional deficiency. The specific nutrients involved include vitamins A, B_{12}, and F, along with manganese. Vitamin A promotes tissue reparation and, subsequently, cellular health. Vitamin B_{12} regulates cell life within a healthy nervous system to keep everything functioning properly. Vitamin F promotes vital organ respiration, and manganese promotes individual tissue respiration. All these functions combine to keep the smaller passageways of the lungs in proper operating condition.

Dosage: You need 5,000 IU of vitamin A and 3 mcg of vitamin B_{12} daily. Vitamin F (unsaturated fatty acids) should make up 10 percent of your total daily calories. You also need 2-5 mg of manganese a day.

Food Sources: Vitamin A comes from green and yellow fruits and vegetables (apricots, spinach, and raw carrots, e.g.), milk, fish liver oil, and beef liver. Vitamin B_{12} is found in cheese, fish, milk, organ meats, and eggs. Vitamin F occurs in vegetable oils, wheat germ, and sunflower seeds. Manganese is supplied by bananas, bran, celery, cereals, egg yolks, green leafy vegetables, legumes, liver, nuts, pineapples, and whole grains.

Atherosclerosis

Description: Atherosclerosis is one of several cardiovascular diseases. This particular condition is best known as "hardening of the arteries," and it is characterized by the formation of plaque on the artery walls.

Recent evidence has revealed that this condition may be due to a deficiency in vitamin B_6 and chromium. B_6 is involved in nerve transmission and tends to facilitate the bodily processes necessary for plaque removal. Chromium increases glucose metabolism, and since fat "burns" in the presence of glucose, more fat will be used rather than deposited on the artery walls.

Dosage: It is recommended that B_6 be taken in amounts of 1.8-2.2 mg and chromium in amounts of .05-.2 mg.

Food Sources: Vitamin B_6 and chromium can be found in similar foods, such as brewer's yeast and whole grain cereals. Additionally, B_6 is supplied by blackstrap molasses, green leafy vegetables, meat, and wheat germ.

Athlete's Foot

Description: Athlete's foot is a contagious infection of the foot caused by a fungus that grows in wet, warm places. There are lesions and blisters between the toes and scaling of the skin. If untreated, the condition can spread to other parts of the body, where a rash and infection can occur. The usual treatment is proper foot care, including washing and drying the feet and applying a medicated powder. Vitamin A has also been used in treatment because it increases the body's resistance to infection as well as helps the body grow new, healthy tissues. It is also possible that a deficiency of vitamin A can increase the susceptibility of an individual to the athlete's foot fungus.

Dosage: You need 5,000 IU of vitamin A daily.

Food Sources: Vitamin A is found in green and yellow fruits and vegetables (apricots, spinach, and raw carrots, e.g.), milk, fish liver oil, and beef liver.

Backache

Description: Pain in the back, usually low-back pain, can result from many causes. The most common include incorrectly lifting a heavy object or sleeping on a bed that is too soft. Sometimes a deficiency of vitamin C can increase susceptibility to backaches. Vitamin C is responsible for collagen production, which is the supporting tissue between bones. A lack of the vitamin leads to an insufficient amount of collagen, which in turn causes a weak and sometimes painful back.

Other sources of back pain include slipped discs, disc fusion, or injury. Back problems should receive medical attention immediately.

Nutritional therapy may be included as part of the treatment, but it should never be the sole treatment.

Dosage: You need 60 mg of vitamin C daily.

Food Sources: Vitamin C is supplied by citrus fruits, cantaloupe, broccoli, green peppers, and potatoes.

Baldness

Description: The loss of hair is most often hereditary, but it can also be due to an illness. Most episodes of baldness occur on the scalp, but other parts of the body may be affected as well. Baldness, in general, is the result of aging, emotional and hormonal factors, and even medication. Baldness may also be caused by a lack of vitamin B complex, C, E, and F. The combination of these vitamins promotes metabolism, energy production, and circulation for cell growth (*read* new hair). Adequate intake of these vitamins may not prevent hereditary baldness, but it may delay its onset.

Dosage: The required dosage of the B complex vitamins varies with each individual vitamin. (See the chart in the appendix.) You should have at least 60 mg of vitamin C a day and 12–15 IU of vitamin E. At least 10 percent of your daily calories should come from unsaturated fatty acids (vitamin F).

Food Sources: The basic sources of the B complex vitamin include blackstrap molasses, brewer's yeast, liver, wheat germ, and whole grains. Vitamin C comes from citrus fruits, cantaloupe, green peppers, broccoli, and potatoes. Vitamin E is found in dark green vegetables, eggs, liver, organ meats, wheat germ, vegetable oils, oatmeal, and tomatoes. You get vitamin F from vegetable oils, wheat germ, and sunflower seeds.

Bedsores
(Decubitus Ulcers)

Description: A bedsore is a serious condition resulting from unrelieved pressure caused by lying in one position for a prolonged period of time. The pressure reduces the blood supply to an area, usually around the bony points of the body, and the soft tissue and skin begin to break down. If the pressure continues, local skin redness occurs, followed by the skin's turning hard and developing a bluish tinge. Eventually, an ulcer will develop and the bone may even become exposed.

Bedsores usually occur in persons who are seriously ill or injured. If they cannot change position on their own, someone should repeatedly move them in a slow and gentle manner. Vitamin C can also help as a treatment because this nutrient promotes red blood cell formation and healing.

Dosage: You should have 60 mg of vitamin C daily.

Food Sources: Vitamin C is supplied by citrus fruits, cantaloupe, broccoli, green peppers, and potatoes.

Beriberi

Description: This is a rare disease of the peripheral nervous system caused by a deficiency of vitamin B_1. The condition is characterized as subclinical beriberi if the symptoms include fatigue, weight loss, appetite suppression, stomach upset, poor reflexes, weakness, memory loss, irritability, and/or depression. It becomes clinical beriberi when pain (neuritis), paralysis of the extremities, cardiovascular changes, edema (swelling), and mental and motor dysfunctions also occur. Proper intake of vitamin B_1 prevents this condition because the vitamin functions to improve appetite, regulate carbohydrate metabolism for energy, and control the transmission of neural impulses between cells.

Dosage: You should have 1–1.5 mg of vitamin B_1 daily.

Food Sources: Vitamin B_1 is found in blackstrap molasses, brewer's yeast, brown rice, fish, meat, nuts, organ meats, poultry, wheat germ, and sunflower seeds.

Bleeding Gums

Description: This symptom is characterized by a weakness in the gums that leads to bleeding whenever external pressure, such as brushing, is applied. A lack of vitamin C is a contributing factor to this condition. However, when sufficient amounts of vitamin C are taken, the problem can be alleviated. This is because vitamin C promotes healing by increasing the strength of cellular tissues and the production of red blood cells. (Note: If this problem persists, see your dentist.)

Dosage: A minimum of 60 mg of vitamin C should be ingested every day.

Food Sources: Vitamin C is found mainly in citrus fruits, cantaloupe, green peppers, broccoli, and potatoes.

Bleeding Stomach Ulcer

Description: An ulcer is an open sore or a lesion. In this case, the ulcer exists in the stomach wall and results in internal bleeding. A deficiency of choline tends to increase the probability of an ulcer's acting up. However, choline serves many functions, mainly in the regulation of fat content in the body. Since protein, not fat, causes acid to be released in the stomach, the combination of all of choline's functions decreases the acid content of the stomach through either absorption or control of the release.

Dosage: There is no specific recommendation for a daily requirement of choline.

Food Sources: Choline is found in brewer's yeast, fish, legumes, organ meats, soybeans, wheat germ, lecithin, egg yolks, and peanuts.

Blemishes

Description: Less serious than acne (but nonetheless a problem), this discoloration of the skin is caused by a lack of vitamin A. Vitamin A can alleviate the problem through its effect on tissue repair and cell growth. New cells grow back and produce the proper skin color.

Dosage: A minimum of 5,000 IU of vitamin A should be ingested daily.

Food Sources: Vitamin A can be found in green and yellow vegetables (spinach and raw carrots, e.g.), and fruits, milk, and fish liver oil.

Body Odor

Description: The noxious smell that emanates from an individual can be due to dirt, germs, or sweat. Often, body odor results from a deficiency of vitamin B_{12}. This vitamin facilitates metabolic processes and nervous system health. These combined functions prevent noxious odors from building up within the body because all potential causes are excreted properly.

Dosage: You need 3 mcg of vitamin B_{12} a day.

Food Sources: Vitamin B_{12} is found in cheese, fish, milk, organ meats, and eggs.

Brittle Nails

Description: This is a condition in which nails just seem to keep splitting and breaking off. The common remedy is to rub oil on the nails, which is supposed to strengthen them. Surprisingly, it works. Nails become stronger and break less easily. The cure actually helps point out a possible cause of brittle nails. A nutritional deficiency of vitamin F (unsaturated fatty acids) decreases the resiliency and lubrication of nail cells. An adequate supply of vitamin F helps nails retain these qualities.

Dosage: Approximately 10 percent of your total calories should contain vitamin F. Men often require up to five times more vitamin F than women because of their larger body size.

Food sources: Vitamin F is found in vegetable oils, wheat germ, and sunflower seeds.

Bronchitis

Description: Bronchitis is an inflammation of the bronchii, which are the passageways of the lungs. It is usually an extension of a cold or an upper respiratory infection. Bronchitis has many of the same symptoms as pneumonia, such as coughing, fever, and labored breathing. The condition is usually caused by a viral infection, and it is more likely to occur when there is a deficiency of vitamins A and C. Vitamin A strengthens cells and tissues and makes them more resistant to infection. Vitamin C also increases the body's resistance to infections, especially colds. Thus, adequate intake of vitamins A and C serves a protective and preventive function.

Dosage: You need 5,000 IU of vitamin A and 60 mg of vitamin C a day.

Food Sources: Vitamin A is found in green and yellow fruits and vegetables (apricots, spinach, and raw carrots, e.g.), milk, fish liver oil, and beef liver. Vitamin C comes from citrus fruits, cantaloupe, broccoli, green peppers, and potatoes.

Bruises

Description: A bruise is best described as a "black and blue mark." Medically, a bruise is an injury or a contusion in which the skin is not broken but there is discoloration due to fluid accumulation.

There is nothing that can prevent a bruise from occurring. However, a lack of vitamin C will hinder the recovery process by reducing the formation of red blood cells. Therefore, it is important to have enough vitamin C to promote the healing process.

Dosage: You should have 60 mg of vitamin C daily.

Food Sources: Vitamin C is found in citrus fruits, cantaloupe, green peppers, broccoli, and potatoes.

Burns

Description: Burns are obviously not caused by a nutritional deficiency. However, the healing process can be speeded up by taking adequate doses of para-aminobenzoic acid (PABA) and zinc. PABA regulates blood cell formation, speeding the healing process by promoting the growth of new cells. PABA can also be applied externally to the affected area to promote healing. (PABA is the protective sunscreen used to prevent sunburn in suntan lotions.) Zinc specifically promotes the healing process of burns, though exactly how it works is not yet known.

Dosage: There is no specific internal dosage for PABA, but 10–100 mg is a suggested range. You also need 15 mg of zinc a day.

Food Sources: PABA is found in blackstrap molasses, brewer's yeast, liver, and wheat germ. Zinc is supplied in brewer's yeast, liver, seafood, soybeans, spinach, sunflower seeds, and mushrooms.

Bursitis

Description: Bursitis is the painful inflammation of the bursa, which is a pouch containing a small amount of fluid located at a point of friction, such as a joint. Bursitis occurs when the bursa becomes inflamed and excess fluid accumulates. The condition is usually caused by a strain on an area or a body part, but sometimes the cause is unknown. It is possible that bursitis may result from a nutritional deficiency in specific instances. The nutrients involved are vitamin B_6, which maintains nervous system functioning; vitamin C, which regulates connective tissue formation; and magnesium, which aids in the metabolism of vitamin C. Tendinitis, an inflammation of a tendon, is a similar condition.

Dosage: You should have 1.8–2.2 mg of vitamin B_6, 60 mg of vitamin C, and 300–350 mg of magnesium a day.

Food Sources: Vitamin B_6 is found in blackstrap molasses; brewer's yeast; green, leafy vegetables; meat; organ meats; wheat germ; whole grains; prunes; brown rice; and peas. Vitamin C comes from citrus fruits, cantaloupe, broccoli, green peppers, and potatoes. Magnesium is supplied by bran, honey, green vegetables, nuts, seafood, spinach, bone meal, kelp tablets, and tuna fish.

Cancer

Description: Cancer is not a single disease, but rather a large number of different diseases. These diseases are characterized by cells that repeatedly subdivide in a random, disorderly manner. The uncontrolled growth of these malignant cells forms tumors that crowd out the healthy tissue and interfere with the functioning of vital organs. If the cancer remains unchecked, the vital organs will cease functioning and death will result.

The causes of cancer are still unknown, but there are certain predisposing factors. Cigarette smoking, air pollution, asbestos, radiation, and overexposure to sunlight are some possible causes. Some treatment measures include chemotherapy and nutritional therapy. The vitamins used most often are A and C. Both of these vitamins strengthen the immune system and aid the body's resistance. Sometimes, with adequate doses or even megadoses, cancers have gone into remission. *However, you should not attempt nutritional therapy in place of medical care.*

Dosage: You need 5,000 IU of vitamin A and 60 mg of vitamin C daily.

Food Sources: Vitamin A is found in green and yellow fruits and vegetables (apricots, spinach, raw carrots, etc.), milk, fish liver oil, and beef liver. Vitamin C comes from citrus fruits, cantaloupe, broccoli, green peppers, and potatoes.

Canker Sores

Description: This is a common ailment that usually occurs during times of stress. A canker sore is an ulceration of the mouth and lips and is quite painful. A deficiency of niacin is related to the onset of canker sores, and an appropriate intake of niacin can improve circulation and the metabolic process to promote the healing of canker sores.

Dosage: A dose of 13-18 mg of niacin should be received daily.

Food Sources: Niacin can be found in brewer's yeast, seafood, lean meats, milk, poultry, and roasted peanuts.

Capillary Wall Ruptures

Description: The weakness in the capillary walls that leads to a breakdown is often due to a deficiency of vitamin C. Vitamin C helps build tissues and promotes the healing process by increasing red blood cell production. These functions contribute to strengthening of the capillary walls and prevention of further ruptures.

Dosage: Vitamin C should be taken as a 60 mg daily dosage.

Food Sources: The best food sources for vitamin C include citrus fruits, cantaloupe, green peppers, broccoli, and potatoes.

Cardiac Arrest

Description: The stopping of the heart beat is not normally attributed to a nutritional deficiency. However, when you consider the functions of the B complex vitamins, and the minerals calcium and potassium, you may see why nutritional deficiencies do play a role in cardiac arrest. The B complex vitamins regulate nervous system activity in general. Calcium controls heart rhythm and nervous system transmission rates. Potassium also helps regulate transmission rates as well as controlling the heartbeat. A deficiency of these three nutrients can definitely affect the functioning of the heart.

Dosage: The B complex vitamins each have their own specific dosages, and these are given in the chart in the appendix. You need 800-1400 mg of calcium a day. There is no specific daily dosage for potassium, but 100-300 mg is suggested.

Food Sources: The basic sources for the B complex vitamins include blackstrap molasses, brewer's yeast, liver, wheat germ, and whole grains. Calcium comes from milk, cheese, molasses, yogurt, bone meal, dolomite, almonds, and beef liver. Potassium is found in dates, figs, peaches, tomato juice, blackstrap molasses, peanuts, raisins, seafood, apricots, bananas, potatoes, and green peppers.

Cataracts

Description: This is an eye disorder in which the lens of the eye and/or its capsule becomes opaque. It is characterized by blurred or distorted vision, and it can eventually lead to blindness. Sometimes it is related to a vitamin B_2 deficiency. B_2 is responsible for cell respiration, which improves the cells' functional capabilities. In the case of the eyes, moisture and circulation are kept up and the eyes can function normally.

Dosage: The acceptable dosage of vitamin B_2 is 1.2–1.7 mg daily.

Food Sources: Vitamin B_2 is found in many of the same foods as the other B complex vitamins. These foods include blackstrap molasses, nuts, organ meats, whole grains, and brewer's yeast.

Colds

Description: Colds are the result of an inflammation of the respiratory mucous membrane. Contrary to popular belief, colds are not caused by poor weather conditions. Colds are caused by a viral infection that becomes prominent when resistance is low. One reason for lowered resistance is a lack of vitamin C. A major function of vitamin C is to provide protection against colds, but this is not as a cure after you catch a cold. It is possible that larger doses of vitamin C will help speed the cold through your system, but this is still speculative.

Dosage: A daily intake of 60 mg of vitamin C will provide sufficient resistance to colds.

Food Sources: Vitamin C is found in citrus fruits, cantaloupe, green peppers, broccoli, and potatoes.

Constipation

Description: This very uncomfortable feeling is best described as an inability to "go to the bathroom." A more scientific definition: difficult or infrequent defecation with the passing of unduly hard and dry fecal materials. Constipation is basically the sluggish action of the bowels.

While constipation may be caused by a host of external factors, such as stress or improper diet, it is often caused by an insufficiency of several nutrients. These include the B complex vitamins, inositol, para-aminobenzoic acid (PABA), and potassium. The B complex vitamins are responsible for the maintenance of muscle tone in the gastrointestinal tract as well as the regulation of metabolism. Inositol and PABA also help control metabolism. When metabolism is working properly, food is digested and waste matter is excreted easily. Finally, potassium's role in muscle contractions helps push the waste matter through the system.

Dosage: The B complex vitamins have individual dosage requirements (see the chart in the appendix). There are no stated requirements for inositol, PABA, or potassium, but suggested ranges are given on the chart in the appendix.

Food Sources: Vitamin B complex, inositol, and PABA are

all found in the same foods. These include blackstrap molasses, brewer's yeast, liver, wheat germ, and whole grains. Potassium is found in dates, figs, peaches, tomato juice, blackstrap molasses, peanuts, raisins, seafood, potatoes, green peppers, and sunflower seeds.

Convulsions

Description: Convulsions appear as wild, uncontrolled, thrashing movements. They are actually rapidly alternating contractions and relaxations of muscles that result in irregular movements of the limbs or the entire body. They can lead to loss of consciousness. Convulsions are usually caused by epilepsy, brain disease, asphyxiation, or brain injury. However, a nutritional deficiency of vitamin B_6 may lead to a loss of motor control that culminates in convulsions. Since a primary function of B_6 is to regulate the sodium-potassium balance in the cells, which is a major factor in neuromuscular control, it is easy to see how B_6 may prevent convulsions.

Dosage: You need 1.8–2.2 mg of vitamin B_6 daily.

Food Sources: Vitamin B_6 is found in blackstrap molasses, brewer's yeast, green leafy vegetables, meat, organ meats, wheat germ, whole grains, dessicated liver, brown rice, and peas.

Cystitis

Description: Cystitis is an inflammation of the bladder and one of the most common disorders of the urinary tract. Cystitis is very rarely a primary disease and is often a symptom of some other disturbance in the urinary tract. People become more susceptible to cystitis when their diets lack vitamins A, B complex, C, D, and E. Vitamins A and C enable the body to resist infection, and vitamins D, E, and B complex promote a healthy nervous system. The combined functions help prevent the inflammation.

Dosage: You need 5,000 IU of vitamin A, 60 mg of C, 400 IU of D, and 12–15 IU of E. The B complex vitamins each have specific dosages (see the chart in the appendix).

Food Sources: Vitamin A is found in green and yellow fruits and vegetables (apricots, spinach, raw carrots, etc.), milk, fish liver oil, and beef liver. The best sources of the B complex vitamins include blackstrap molasses, brewer's yeast, liver, wheat germ, and whole grains. Vitamin C comes from citrus fruits, cantaloupe, broccoli, green peppers, and potatoes. Vitamin D is supplied by egg yolks, organ meats, bone meal, sunlight, milk, salmon, and tuna fish. Vitamin E occurs in dark green vegetables, eggs, liver, organ meats, wheat germ, vegetable oils, oatmeal, peanuts, and tomatoes.

Dandruff

Description: Dandruff is simply small flakes of dead skin from the scalp. It is the result of a disturbance in the hair oil glands. When too little oil is produced, the hair becomes dry and brittle and white flakes usually appear. This can occur just because you use a blow dryer too close to your scalp. On the other hand, you may have yellow dandruff, which is due to an excessive production of oil. Either symptom is usually accompanied by itching.

The actual cause of dandruff is not fully understood, but it may be due to a vitamin and mineral deficiency. The nutrients involved are vitamins B_6, B_{12}, and F and selenium. Both B_6 and

B_{12} regulate metabolism and nervous system function. This aids in the nourishment of the hair follicles. Vitamin F promotes glandular activity and cell growth, which leads to a healthy scalp. Selenium is a mineral that works synergistically with vitamin E to facilitate blood circulation. A healthy diet will supply appropriate amounts of these nutrients and, along with frequent hair washings and scalp massages, may be the best cure for dandruff.

Dosage: You need 1.8–2.2 mg of vitamin B_6 and 3 mcg of vitamin B_{12}. About 10 percent of your total calories should supply vitamin F (unsaturated fatty acids). You also need 50–100 mcg of selenium daily.

Food Sources: Vitamin B_6 comes from blackstrap molasses, brewer's yeast, green leafy vegetables, meat, organ meats, wheat germ, whole grains, brown rice, and peas. Vitmain B_{12} is found in cheese, fish, milk, organ meats, and eggs. Vitamin F occurs in vegetable oils, wheat germ, and sunflower seeds. You can get selenium from bran, wheat germ, broccoli, onions, tomatoes, and tuna fish.

Dehydration

Description: This is a condition in which there is excessive water or fluid loss from body tissues without replacement. Common causes of dehydration include overexertion during hot weather, diarrhea, and vomiting. Also, a deficiency of sodium in the body can lead to dehydration. Sodium enables body tissues to retain water, thus slowing or preventing the dehydration process.

One should *not* take salt tablets or drink commercial energy drinks to replace fluids. Drink plenty of water and salt your food, if necessary. These are the safest and most effective methods for managing dehydration.

Dosage: There is no specific daily requirement for sodium, but it is suggested that intake not exceed 2,000 mg a day.

Food Sources: Sodium is supplied by salt, milk, cheese, and seafood.

Dental Cavities

Description: A cavity is a hollow space in a tooth produced by dental caries. Quite often, cavities are caused by the foods we eat, improper brushing, lack of flossing. While it is very difficult to prevent cavities from ever occurring, we can do our best not to encourage them to appear. This involves having an adequate daily supply of vitamins C and D and calcium. All three nutrients promote bone and tooth formation. Thus, strong, healthy, well-nourished teeth will offset the effect of the caries.

Dosage: The daily requirement for vitamin C is 60 mg; for vitamin D, 400 IU; and for calcium, 800–1400 mg.

Food Sources: Vitamin C is found in citrus fruits, cantaloupe, green peppers, broccoli, and potatoes. Vitamin D occurs in egg yolks, organ meats, bone meal, sunlight, milk, salmon, and tuna. Calcium is found in milk, cheese, molasses, yogurt, bone meal, dolomite, almonds, and beef liver.

Depression

Description: This is a psychological condition characterized by emotional feelings of sadness, helplessness, and low self-worth. Depression is often brought about by grief, loss of a loved one, or an inability to accomplish one's goals. Recently, evidence has accumulated that depression may result from nutritional deficiencies. Specifically, the vitamins are B_6, biotin, niacin, and para-aminobenzoic acid (PABA). All these vitamins are involved in nervous system control and the regulation of metabolic processes. This leads to better nourishment of the cells and more effective functioning.

Dosage: Take 1.8-2.2 mg of vitamin B_6 per day. Biotin should be ingested on a daily basis; take 150-300 mcg. You need 13-18 mg of niacin a day. There is no specific recommendation for PABA.

Food Sources: These vitamins are commonly found in such foods as blackstrap molasses, brewer's yeast, whole grains, organ meats, and wheat germ. Additionally, B_6 comes from green leafy vegetables and brown rice; biotin is in legumes and egg yolks, niacin is also found in milk, poultry, and seafood; and PABA can be found in liver.

Dermatitis

Description: This is an inflammation of the skin that can have many causes, including allergic reactions, emotional stress, fatigue, and a deficiency of the B complex vitamins. These vitamins are responsible for metabolism, energy production, cell growth, and nervous system regulation. These functions combine to prevent the skin from flaring up. Additionally, the B complex vitamins help the body control stress and manage fatigue. Thus, the removal of two of the causes of dermatitis obviously lessens the possibility of its occurrence.

Dosage: Each B vitamin has its own specific dosage, which is given in the chart in the appendix.

Food Sources: The basic sources of the B complex vitamins include blackstrap molasses, brewer's yeast, liver, wheat gern, and whole grains.

Diabetes

Description: The cause of this disease is not fully understood, but the condition is simply a breakdown in metabolism. The body is unable to oxidize glucose because of an insufficient supply of insulin. The result is a high level of blood sugar. The likelihood of diabetes is increased when there is a nutritional deficiency of vitamins A, B_1, B_2, and E, and the minerals chromium, potassium, and zinc. All these nutrients aid the body's digestive and metabolic processes, which should enable the pancreas to produce enough insulin to keep the blood sugar levels within normal limits.

Diabetes is an illness that should be cared for under medical supervision. Proper diet and exercise are your responsibility, but do not neglect your physician's role in the treatment of diabetes.

Dosage: You need 5,000 IU of vitamin A, 1-1.5 mg of B_1, 1.3-1.7 mg of B_2, and 12-15 IU of vitamin E a day. You also need .05-.2 mg of chromium and 15 mg of zinc daily. There is no specific dosage for potassium, but the suggested range is 100-300 mg.

Food Sources: Vitamin A comes from green and yellow fruits and vegetables (apricots, spinach, and raw carrots, e.g.), milk, fish liver oil, and beef liver. Vitamin B_1 is found in blackstrap molasses, brewer's yeast, brown rice, fish, meat, nuts, organ meats, poultry, and wheat germ. Vitamin B_2 is supplied by blackstrap molasses, nuts, organ meats, whole grains, Brussels sprouts, and brewer's yeast. Vitamin E occurs in dark green vegetables, eggs, liver, organ meats, wheat germ, vegetable oils, oatmeal, peanuts, and tomatoes. You get chromium from brewer's yeast, clams, corn oil, and whole grain cereals. Potassium is provided by dates, figs, peaches, tomato juice, blackstrap molasses, peanuts, raisins, seafood, apricots, bananas, potatoes, sunflower seeds, and green peppers. Finally, you can find zinc in brewer's yeast, liver, seafood, soybeans, spinach, sunflower seeds, and mushrooms.

Diarrhea

Description: Diarrhea is characterized by frequent passage of abnormally loose and watery bowel movements. Quite often, diarrhea occurs as a reaction to some foods we have eaten. Other times, the digestive system reacts with diarrhea because of a nutritional deficiency of pantothenic acid and vitamins D, F, and K. Pantothenic acid is involved in energy conversion, which improves the functioning of the digestive system. Vitamin D ensures that the nervous system properly activates those muscles and organs responsible for digestion. Vitamins F and K are involved with blood transportation through the system, which leads to appropriate cell nourishment and subsequent function.

Dosage: It is recommended that .5–10 mg of pantothenic acid be ingested daily. While there is a recommendation of 400 IU of vitamin D a day, there is no minimum for vitamins F (10 percent of calories is suggested) and K.

Food Sources: Pantothenic acid is found in brewer's yeast, legumes, organ meats, salmon, wheat germ, orange juice, and whole grains. You can receive vitamin D from egg yolks, organ meats, bone meal, sunlight, milk, salmon, and tuna. Vitamin F is found in vegetable oils, wheat germ, and sunflower seeds. The major sources of vitamin K include green leafy vegetables, safflower oil, blackstrap molasses, yogurt, oatmeal, and beef liver.

Digestive Disturbances

Description: These problems involve a host of factors related to an inability to digest food properly. The results can be excess gas, excess stomach acid, or cramps. Aside from being caused by foods we have eaten, digestive disturbances can result from a nutritional deficiency of the B complex vitamins and vitamin C. The B complex vitamins facilitate metabolic processes and regulate muscle tone in the digestive system. Vitamin C helps the digestive process and also allows other vitamins to do their job.

Dosage: The daily intake of the B complex vitamins varies with each individual vitamin. The recommended amounts are given on the chart in the appendix. At least 60 mg of vitamin C should be taken daily.

Food Sources: The B complex vitamins are found in blackstrap molasses, brewer's yeast, liver, and whole grains. Vitamin C comes from citrus fruits, cantaloupe, green peppers, broccoli, and potatoes.

Dizziness

Description: Dizziness is a sensation of whirling or the feeling that you are going to fall. People often describe it as feeling woozy or as if the room is spinning around. While a blow to the head or fluid imbalance in the inner ear can lead to dizziness, it can also be caused by a deficiency of vitamins B_2 and B_6. B_2 is involved with cell respiration, which leads to proper cell functioning. B_6 helps regulate the functioning of the nervous system. The combination of these functions leads to greater balance control.

Dosage: You should have 1.3–1.7 mg of vitamin B_2 a day and 1.8–2.2 mg of B_6.

Food Sources: Both vitamins are found in blackstrap molasses, brewer's yeast, nuts, whole grains, green leafy vegetables, and organ meats.

Drowsiness

Description: Drowsiness is a feeling of tiredness or sleepiness. In many instances lack of sleep or overexertion can cause drowsiness. It can also be caused by an insufficient supply of biotin, a B complex vitamin. Biotin promotes metabolism to provide energy. Biotin also facilitates the body's utilization of the other B complex vitamins to promote a properly functioning nervous system and energy production. As long as the body has enough energy to perform its tasks, drowsiness will not occur.

Dosage: You should have 150–300 mcg of biotin a day.

Food Sources: Biotin comes from legumes, whole grains, organ meats, brewer's yeast, egg yolks, beef liver, and soybeans.

Dry Hair

Description: When hair lacks the appropriate nutrients it tends to become dry, coarse, and, at times, brittle. The problem is due to a deficiency in several vitamins. These include vitamins A, B complex, E, and F and the mineral iodine. Vitamin A is involved in tissue repair, so new cells can grow and retain the appropriate amount of moisture. The B complex vitamins and iodine are responsible for aiding metabolism, which in turn nourishes the cells. Vitamin E increases blood flow, and vitamin F promotes growth and vital organ respiration. All these vitamins and iodine combine to facilitate the growth of healthy hair follicles.

Dosage: You should have 5,000 IU of vitamin A a day, 12–15 IU of E, and 100–130 mcg of iodine. Vitamin F should make up 10 percent of your caloric consumption. The B complex vitamins each require different dosages, given on the chart in the appendix.

Food Sources: The best sources of vitamin A are green and yellow fruits and vegetables (spinach and raw carrots, e.g.), milk, and fish liver oil. Vitamin B complex is found in blackstrap molasses, brewer's yeast, liver, and whole grains. Sources of vitamin E include dark green vegetables, eggs, liver, organ meats, wheat germ, vegetable oils, oatmeal, peanuts, and tomatoes. Vitamin F comes from vegetable oils, wheat germ, and sunflower seeds. Iodine occurs in seafood, kelp tablets, and iodized salt.

Duodenal Ulcers

Description: These are open sores or lesions in the duodenum (intestine) that usually result from an oversecretion of gastric juices. The only thing that can be done nutritionally about this problem is to improve the digestive process. Pantothenic acid does this by facilitating metabolism and energy conversion, thereby decreasing the release of excessive gastric juices into the system.

Dosage: From .5 to 10 mg of pantothenic acid should be taken daily.

Food Sources: Pantothenic acid is found in brewer's yeast, legumes, organ meats, salmon, wheat germ, whole grains, and fresh orange juice.

Eczema

Description: This skin condition is characterized by an acute or chronic inflammation that is associated with scales, crusts, or scabs. Many people believe eczema is the result of constant scratching, but more often than not it is due to a lack of inositol, pantothenic acid, and vitamin F. All of these vitamins are involved in the regulation of metabolic processes, the result of which is the growth of new and healthy skin cells.

Dosage: Only pantothenic acid has a recommended daily dosage, which is .5-10 mg. It is suggested that vitamin F make up 10 percent of your total calories. There is no specific recommendation for inositol.

Food Sources: Inositol is found in blackstrap molasses, citrus fruits, brewer's yeast, meat, milk, nuts, vegetables, whole grains, and lecithin. Pantothenic acid occurs in brewer's yeast, legumes, organ meats, salmon, wheat germ, whole grains, and fresh orange juice. Vitamin F comes from vegetable oils, wheat germ, and sunflower seeds.

Edema

Description: Edema is swelling due to retention of fluids. It usually occurs in women just prior to their menstrual periods. Edema is also the result of too much sodium, a mineral that tends to cause the body to hold water. While the condition is not caused by a vitamin deficiency, edema can be regulated and possibly overcome through adequate intake of vitamin B_6. A major function of this vitamin is to maintain the sodium-potassium balance in the system. Therefore, if excess sodium is not present, excess fluid cannot accumulate.

Dosage: A dose of 1.8–2.2 mg of vitamin B_6 is needed daily.

Food Sources: Vitamin B_6 comes from blackstrap molasses, brewer's yeast, green leafy vegetables, meat, organ meats, wheat germ, whole grains, prunes, brown rice, and peas.

Emotional Instability

Description: A person who lacks control over emotional reactions, or who is extremely volatile in his or her reactions, is usually suffering from an inordinate amount of stress. However, it is also possible that the emotional instability is due to a lack of vitamin B_1. This vitamin helps regulate both the nervous system and the digestive system. Thus, proper neural connections are made, and the brain cells receive sufficient nourishment. The lability of the emotional reactions can then eventually be stabilized. *Be aware, though, that adequate amounts of vitamin B_1 do not guarantee a cure for this problem. Professional therapeutic help may be necessary.*

Dosage: You need 1–1.5 mg of vitamin B_1 daily.

Food Sources: Vitamin B_1 is found in blackstrap molasses, brewer's yeast, brown rice, fish, meat, nuts, organ meats, poultry, and wheat germ.

Fatigue

Description: The sensation of fatigue is characterized by feelings of listlessness, tiredness, weariness, and a general lack of energy. Fatigue is often caused by insufficient rest and sometimes by overexertion. Many times, however, fatigue is a result of nutritional deficiencies. The essential nutrients include vitamins A and B complex, phosphorus, and zinc. All these vitamins and minerals help facilitate the metabolic processes of the body. This enhances energy conversion and muscular activity. Thus, feelings of fatigue give way to feelings of vigor.

Dosage: You should have 5,000 IU of vitamin A daily, along with 800 mg of phosphorus and 15 mg of zinc. The B complex vitamins should be taken in specific amounts for each vitamin (see the chart in the appendix).

Food Sources: Vitamin A is found in green and yellow fruits and vegetables (spinach and raw carrots, e.g.), milk, and fish liver oil. Vitamin B complex occurs in blackstrap molasses, brewer's yeast, liver, and whole grains. Good sources of phosphorus include eggs, fish, grains, meat, poultry, yellow cheese, and yogurt. You will find zinc in brewer's yeast, liver, seafood, soybeans, spinach, sunflower seeds, and mushrooms.

Gallstones

Description: Gallstones are concretions (rocklike substances) found in the gallbladder or bile ducts. They are usually caused by insufficient metabolism of fats. Vitamin F prevents the formation of gallstones by aiding in circulation and glandular activity and reducing cholesterol. These factors decrease the chances of a concretion being formed.

Dosage: There is no stated recommended dosage for vitamin F, but you should consume at least 10 percent of your total calories in unsaturated fatty acids.

Food Sources: Vitamin F is found in vegetable oils, wheat germ, and sunflower seeds.

Gastritis

Description: Gastritis is basically an inflammation of the stomach. In its acute form gastritis can be caused by an infection, overeating, medication, or drinking too much alcohol. Chronic gastritis is usually the result of a long-term irritant, ulcers, repeated emotional upsets, or a vitamin deficiency in B complex and C. The B complex vitamins help regulate metabolism, energy production, and the muscle tone of the gastrointestinal tract. Vitamin C also aids in the digestive process. Together, these vitamins prevent the stomach from becoming irritated and inflamed.

Dosage: The required dosage of the B complex vitamins varies with the individual vitamins (see the chart in the appendix). You need 60 mg of vitamin C daily.

Food Sources: The basic sources of the B complex vitamins include blackstrap molasses, brewer's yeast, liver, wheat germ, and whole grains. You can get vitamin C from citrus fruits, cantaloupe, green peppers, broccoli, and potatoes.

Gingivitis

Description: Gingivitis is an inflammation of the gums (gingiva) that begins with a slight swelling along the gum margin of one or more teeth. There may be some discoloration. As the condition worsens, the gum separates from the tooth surface, but there is no pain. The gum tissue may even bleed with slight pressure. Gingivitis is usually caused by a deficiency in vitamin C. The condition can also be a precursor to scurvy.

Vitamin C is responsible for bone and tooth formation, collagen (connective tissue) production, red blood cell formation, and tissue repair. It is easy to see how all these functions serve to prevent gingivitis.

Dosage: You need 60 mg of vitamin C daily.

Food Sources: Vitamin C comes from citrus fruits, cantaloupe, broccoli, green peppers, and tomatoes.

Glucose Intolerance (in Diabetics)

Description: This symptom refers to the inability to metabolize glucose. Genetics and insulin production are responsible for this problem, but glucose intolerance is also related to a deficiency of chromium. This mineral helps regulate blood sugar levels and glucose metabolism for energy production.

Dosage: The daily requirement for chromium is .05–.2 mg.

Food Sources: Chromium is found in brewer's yeast, clams, corn oil, and whole grain cereals.

Gray Hair

Description: The change from natural hair color to gray is often thought to be simply a by-product of aging. If that were always true, every elderly person would have gray hair. Since not everyone has or gets gray hair, there must be another cause. A nutritional deficiency of folic acid and para-aminobenzoic acid (PABA) can also lead to gray hair. Folic acid regulates protein metabolism, and hair is protein. PABA is directly involved with hair color and its restoration, along with protein metabolism. Thus, it is easy to see how these two nutrients can help you maintain or possibly regain your original hair color.

Dosage: You should have 400 mcg of folic acid a day. There is no recommendation for the daily intake of PABA.

Food Sources: Folic acid is found in green leafy vegetables (such as spinach), milk, organ meats, oysters, salmon, whole grains, brewer's yeast, and tuna fish. PABA comes from black-strap molasses, brewer's yeast, liver, organ meats, and wheat germ.

Growth Problems

Description: Disturbances in maturational growth and development are often attributed to a dysfunctional pituitary gland. Recent research indicates that nutritional deficiencies also play a role in growth problems. Specifically, a lack of vitamin B_2, folic acid, choline, and zinc is responsible for growth disturbances. Vitamin B_2 helps regulate cellular function and metabolism, both of which contribute to proper growth. Folic acid is directly involved in body growth, while choline is indirectly involved through the regulation of nerve transmission. Finally, zinc helps regulate digestion, metabolism, and the growth of various body organs. The seemingly diverse functions of these nutrients combine to promote proper growth and development.

Dosage: You should have 1.3–1.7 mg of vitamin B_2 per day, 400 mcg of folic acid, and 15 mg of zinc. There is no specified daily amount for choline.

Food Sources: Vitamin B_2 is found in blackstrap molasses, nuts, organ meats, whole grains, and brewer's yeast. Folic acid comes from green leafy vegetables (such as spinach), milk, organ meats, oysters, salmon, whole grains, brewer's yeast, and tuna fish. Choline is found in brewer's yeast, fish, legumes, organ meats, soybeans, wheat germ, lecithin, egg yolks, and peanuts. The best sources of zinc include brewer's yeast, liver, seafood, soybeans, spinach, sunflower seeds, and mushrooms. It is obvious that many of the same foods supply all these nutrients, so a well-balanced diet should overcome any deficiencies and facilitate growth.

Halitosis

Description: This is the scientific term for bad breath. The problem can be alleviated by brushing or rinsing (gargling) with a mouthwash regularly to rid the mouth of germs. However, the symptom is usually the result of food repeating from the stomach. This repetition is caused by improper production of hydrochloric acid and improper function of the metabolism. Niacin regulates both these functions and, when taken in proper amounts, will often cure the problem.

Dosage: You should have from 13–18 mg of niacin daily.

Food Sources: The best sources of niacin are brewer's yeast, seafood, lean meats, poultry, and dessicated liver.

Hay Fever

Description: *Hay fever* is the popular term for allergic rhinitis, which is an inflammation inside the nose due to an allergy. The symptoms resemble those of a cold, but there is no fever. The mucous membrane in the nose and eyelids becomes puffed up; there is sneezing and a watery discharge from the eyes and nose. Hay fever is caused by allergens such as pollen, animal fur, feathers, and household dust. It is also possible that a nutritional deficiency of the vitamin B complex and vitamins C and E may make a person more susceptible to hay fever. Additionally, adequate intake of these nutrients, along with conventional medical treatment, should help relieve the problem.

The B complex vitamins, along with vitamin C, help regulate metabolism and the nervous system. Vitamin E improves circulation. Together, these nutrients keep the body strong and able to ward off the allergens.

Dosage: The B complex vitamins each have their own individual doses (see the chart in the appendix). You also need 60 mg of vitamin C and 12–15 IU of vitamin E daily.

Food Sources: The basic food sources of the B complex vitamins include brewer's yeast, blackstrap molasses, liver, wheat germ, and whole grains. Vitamin C is supplied by citrus fruits, cantaloupe, broccoli, green peppers, and potatoes. Vitamin E comes from dark green vegetables, eggs, liver, organ meats, wheat germ, vegetables, oatmeal, peanuts, and tomatoes.

Headaches

Description: Throbbing or aching in the head is usually the result of stress and tension. Quite often, headaches can also be caused by what you eat or do not eat. While the causes of headaches vary, and the type and location of the pain also vary, the cure always seems to be the same: aspirin. However, the headache may be caused by a deficiency of niacin and para-aminobenzoic acid (PABA) in the system. Niacin regulates circulation, which will control the flow of blood to the brain and ease the pain. PABA contributes indirectly through its effect on blood cell formation.

Dosage: There is no daily recommendation for PABA, but you should have 13–18 mg of niacin.

Food Sources: Niacin and PABA are found in such foods as brewer's yeast, blackstrap molasses, liver, and wheat germ.

Heart Disease

Description: There is no known *cure* for any type of heart disease, but there are several recommended ways to reduce the risk. Exercise, stress management, and proper diet are among the most popular and the most controllable of these risk reduction methods. It is also possible to lessen the risk of heart disease through ingestion of the proper combination of vitamins and minerals—specifically, vitamins B_{15} (pangamic acid), C, and E, niacin, choline, inositol, and calcium. Vitamin B_{15} is involved with cell oxidation, which helps build strong and healthy cells. Niacin regulates circulation and reduces the level of cholesterol. Choline aids in fat metabolism and the formation of lecithin, which is an emulsifier. Inositol also aids in the production of lecithin and simultaneously reduces cholesterol. This prevents hardening of the arteries. Vitamin C serves a general healing and protective function in the body. Vitamin E reduces cholesterol, acts as an anticlotting factor, and increases the blood flow to the heart. Calcium regulates nerve transmission and, subsequently, heart rate. Taken together, these nutrients may provide a protective barrier against heart disease. However, you should always remember that many other factors must be considered.

Dosage: There are no recommended daily dosages for vitamin B_{15}, choline, or inositol. You should have 13–19 mg of niacin a day, 60 mg of vitamin C, 12–15 IU of vitamin E, and 800–1,400 mg of calcium.

Food Sources: Vitamin B_{15} occurs naturally in brewer's yeast, brown rice, rare meat, seeds, whole grains, and organ meats. Niacin is found in brewer's yeast, seafood, lean meats, poultry, milk, and dessicated liver. Choline comes from brewer's yeast, fish, legumes, organ meats, soybeans, wheat germ, lecithin, egg yolks, and peanuts. Inositol is found in blackstrap molasses, citrus fruits, brewer's yeast, meat, milk, nuts, vegetables, and whole grains. The best sources of vitamin C include citrus fruits, cantaloupe, green peppers, broccoli, and potatoes. Vitamin E can be found in dark green vegetables, eggs, liver, wheat germ, vegetable oils, oatmeal, and tomatoes. You can get calcium from milk, cheese, molasses, yogurt, bone meal, dolomite, almonds, and beef liver.

Heart Palpitations

Description: You may feel a throbbing, thumping, excessive, or skipped beating of your heart, which can come from several causes. Stress and a dysfunction of the heart's natural pacemaker are two possibilities. Whatever the cause, palpitations can usually be controlled by ingesting sufficient amounts of calcium. This mineral regulates heart rhythm through its control of nerve transmission.

Dosage: You need between 800 and 1,400 mg of calcium per day.

Food Sources: The best sources of calcium include milk, cheese, molasses, yogurt, bone meal, dolomite, almonds, and beef liver.

Hemorrhaging

Description: Hemorrhaging is a condition of excessive bleeding that can occur either externally or internally. It is also known as *hypoprothrombinemia,* which is defined as a tendency to bleed. The condition can result from a lack of vitamin K, whose primary function is to promote blood clotting. When vitamin K is deficient, external wounds continue to bleed; internal bleeding is evidenced when blood is coughed up or excreted in the urine or feces. A lack of vitamin C, which aids in the formation of red blood cells, can also lead to hemorrhaging.

Dosage: There is no recommended daily dosage for vitamin K, but it is thought that 300–500 mcg might be sufficient to prevent a deficiency. You also need 60 mg of vitamin C a day.

Food Sources: Vitamin K is found in green leafy vegetables, safflower oil, blackstrap molasses, yogurt, oatmeal, and liver. Vitmain C comes from citrus fruits, cantaloupe, green peppers, broccoli, and potatoes.

Hepatitis

Description: Hepatitis is an inflammation of the liver, usually caused by a viral infection. The condition can be either infectious hepatitis, which is spread by food or water that has been contaminated by the feces of carriers, or serum hepatitis, which is spread by blood transfusions from infected donors. There is an incubation period for both types of hepatitis. After this period has passed, the symptoms of viral hepatitis develop suddenly. These include loss of appetite, fever, nausea, and pain or tenderness in the upper right portion of the abdomen. The urine may become dark due to bile pigments. Medical treatment must be sought. Along with bed rest and gamma globulin injections, vitamin C may also be used. This nutrient promotes both the healing process and the formation of red blood cells. Both of these functions would strengthen the body's ability to fight off the infection. Additionally, vitamin C helps the body resist infection, and adequate or even megadoses may prevent this illness from occurring.

Dosage: You need 60 mg of vitamin C daily.

Food Sources: Vitamin C is supplied by citrus fruits, cantaloupe, broccoli, green peppers, and potatoes.

High Cholesterol Level

Description: Cholesterol is a fatlike substance that is both manufactured in and ingested into the body. It is a normal constituent of bile, and it serves many positive functions. However, most people are aware of cholesterol because of its relation to heart disease. While high cholesterol levels in the blood are often caused by the foods we eat, these levels are also affected by the amount of vitamin F and inositol we take in. Vitamin F refers to unsaturated fatty acids that help reduce cholesterol levels and prevent plaque buildup. Inositol also reduces cholesterol levels and retards the artery-hardening process. Additionally, inositol aids in the formation of lecithin, which is an emulsifying agent that promotes the metabolism of fat and cholesterol. Therefore, while a high cholesterol level cannot be *cured* with vitamins, it can certainly be reduced and/or prevented.

Dosage: There is no recommended daily dosage for either of these nutrients, but unsaturated fatty acids should make up 10 percent of your total calories.

Food Sources: Vitamin F is found in vegetable oils, wheat germ, and sunflower seeds. Inositol is found in blackstrap molasses, citrus fruits, brewer's yeast, meat, milk, nuts, vegetables, and whole grains.

Hypertension (High Blood Pressure)

Description: Blood pressure is considered high when the reading is greater than 140/90. Many factors can cause hypertension: stress, diet, genetics, heart disease, obesity, and lack of exercise. Modifications in these factors, except genetics, can reduce blood pressure readings. Proper nutrient supplementation can also lower blood pressure.

While the necessary nutrients are the same as for heart disease, choline seems to have a greater effect on blood pressure than any of the others. Perhaps this is because choline is involved with the regulation of metabolism and nerve transmission, which subsequently leads to proper functioning of the circulatory system.

Dosage: There is no specific daily recommendation for choline.

Food Sources: Choline is found in brewer's yeast, fish, legumes, organ meats, soybeans, wheat germ, lecithin, egg yolks, and peanuts.

Hypoglycemia

Description: This is low blood sugar, and it is characterized by acute fatigue, restlessness, irritability, and weakness. Hypoglycemia is the result of an excess of insulin. One nutrient that may be lacking in a hypoglycemic is pantothenic acid, which is involved in energy conversion. Glucose is the body's primary source of energy. Pantothenic acid regulates the conversion of glucose to energy. Thus, the blood sugar levels will remain stable.

Dosage: You need a minimum of .5–10 mg of pantothenic acid per day.

Food Sources: Pantothenic acid is found in brewer's yeast, legumes, organ meats, salmon, wheat germ, whole grains, and fresh orange juice.

Hypothyroidism
(Goiter)

Description: This is a condition in which the thyroid gland produces too little of its hormone, thyroxine. The cause is often a nutritional deficiency of vitamin D and iodine. If these nutrients are not received in adequate supply, you may become lethargic and have a tendency to put on weight. Eventually, the thyroid gland becomes enlarged because of its efforts to produce thyroxine. The typical treatment is to give the patient thyroxine, but adequate amounts of vitamin D and iodine, taken regularly, can keep the thyroid gland functioning properly. This is because of their effects on the nervous system and metabolism, and their secondary effects on the circulatory system. All these functions combine to stimulate the thyroid gland to produce thyroxine.

Dosage: You need 400 IU of vitamin D and 100–130 mcg of iodine daily.

Food Sources: Vitamin D comes from egg yolks, organ meats, bone meal, sunlight, milk, salmon, and tuna fish. Iodine is supplied by seafood, kelp tablets, and iodized salt.

Hysteria

Description: Hysteria is a condition in which an individual shows uncontrollable emotions (such as excessive laughing or crying) and a wild flailing of the limbs. Hysteria is usually a reaction to an unbearable situation, and this type of behavior usually serves as an escape.

The hysterical reaction usually wears itself out, but when it does not, or it recurs continuously, the best treatment is psychotherapy. One approach within psychotherapy has been to consider a nutritional deficiency of the B complex vitamins, specifically B_6. Vitamin B_6 helps maintain the proper functioning of the nervous system. This could possibly prevent overexcitability and hysterical reactions.

Dosage: Vitamin B_6 should be taken in 1.8–2.2 mg doses daily.

Food Sources: Vitamin B_6 is found in blackstrap molasses, brewer's yeast, green leafy vegetables, meat, organ meats, wheat germ, whole grains, prunes, brown rice, and peas.

Impotence

Description: This is the inability of a man to achieve or maintain an erection. Impotence can be caused by physical or emotional trauma or a nutritional deficiency of vitamin E. Vitamin E has often been called the "sex vitamin" because it specifically improves male potency. This probably results from vitamin E's positive effect on circulation.

Dosage: You should take 12–15 IU of vitamin E daily.

Food Sources: The best sources of vitamin E include dark green vegetables, eggs, liver, wheat germ, vegetable oils, oatmeal, and tomatoes.

Indigestion (Dyspepsia)

Description: *Indigestion* is the term usually given to describe disturbances in the digestive system. These include nausea, vomiting, stomachache or abdominal cramps, belching, or feelings of fullness. Indigestion can have many causes, such as emotional upset, overeating, eating too fast, or eating foods that do not agree with you. Indigestion may also be a result of a vitamin B_1 and B_2 deficiency. Both these vitamins regulate metabolic and digestive processes, enabling food to be transported properly through the digestive system.

Dosage: You need 1–1.5 mg of vitamin B_1 and 1.3–1.7 mg of vitamin B_2 daily.

Food Sources: Vitamin B_1 comes from blackstrap molasses, brewer's yeast, brown rice, fish, meat, nuts, organ meats, poultry, and wheat germ. Vitamin B_2 is found in blackstrap molasses, nuts, organ meats, whole grains, brewer's yeast, and Brussels sprouts.

Infertility

Description: This condition is the same as sterility. It refers most often to the inability of a female to become pregnant, but it also describes the inability of a male to impregnate a female. The cause may be an organic or a functional defect. At other times infertility can be caused by a lack of vitamin E and zinc. Vitamin E directly promotes fertility and male potency, and zinc is responsible for reproductive and sexual organ growth and development.

Dosage: You need 12–15 IU of vitamin E and 15 mg of zinc a day.

Food Sources: Vitamin E is supplied by dark green vegetables, eggs, liver, organ meats, wheat germ, vegetable oils, oatmeal, peanuts, and tomatoes. Zinc is found in brewer's yeast, liver, seafood, soybeans, spinach, sunflower seeds, and mushrooms.

Insomnia

Description: Insomia is a common problem among elderly people or people who are under a great deal of stress. These individuals find it difficult to fall asleep or find themselves continually waking up. Thus, their sleep periods are constantly interrupted. In addition to insomnia induced by external causes, people can have sleep problems because of nutritional deficiencies. A lack of vitamin B complex, vitamin D, and calcium can lead to sleeplessness. All these nutrients, when taken in sufficient amounts, combine to regulate nervous system activity. Essentially, the transmission rates of the nerve impulses are slowed down, and this results in less interrupted sleep.

Dosage: The dosage for the B complex vitamins varies with each vitamin (see the chart in the appendix for the recommended ranges). You should have 400 IU of vitamin D a day, along with 800–1,400 mg of calcium.

Food Sources: The B complex vitamins are found in brewer's yeast, blackstrap molasses, liver, whole grains, and legumes. Vitamin D comes from egg yolks, organ meats, sunlight, bone meal, milk, salmon, and tuna. You get calcium in milk, cheese, molasses, yogurt, bone meal, dolomite, almonds, and beef liver.

Intestinal Disorders

Description: These disorders involve a general inability of the intestines to complete the digestive process. Often, the result is constipation, cramps, diarrhea, or excessive gas. While reactions to certain foods may cause intestinal problems, they are also related to a deficiency of pantothenic acid. This nutrient is responsible for the regulation of energy conversion in the digestive system, which leads to a reduction of intestinal dysfunction.

Dosage: You should have between .5 and 10 mg of pantothenic acid per day.

Food Sources: Pantothenic acid is found in brewer's yeast, legumes, organ meats, salmon, wheat germ, whole grains, and orange juice.

Intestinal Gas

Description: This is a specific intestinal disorder that results when excessive nitrogenous waste products are trapped in this section of the digestive tract. Reactions to foods may be partially responsible, but a lack of sodium also contributes to this disorder. Sodium helps the body maintain normal cellular fluid levels for proper functioning, and regulates the muscle contraction process. These functions, when related specifically to the lower gastrointestinal tract, will help the intestines perform more efficiently without trapping gas.

Dosage: There is no recommended daily dosage of sodium, but it has been suggested that intake be limited to 2,000 mg per day and that no salt be added to foods.

Food Sources: Sodium is found in salt, milk, cheese, seafood, and cured meat products, along with many other types of foods.

Irritability

Description: People become irritable and overreact in a negative fashion for many reasons. Some of the more common causes include dieting, stress, and lack of sleep. A less well-known cause is a deficiency of vitamin B_1. This vitamin helps regulate many of the digestive and metabolic processes, along with blood circulation and energy production. Obviously, a well-fed and properly functioning body will not be so hypersensitive in its response to external influences.

Dosage: You should have 1–1.5 mg of vitamin B_1 daily.

Food Sources: Vitamin B_1 is found in blackstrap molasses, brewer's yeast, brown rice, fish, meat, nuts, poultry, and wheat germ.

Itching/Burning Eyes

Description: This feeling is due to some type of irritation that causes you to want to rub or scratch the eyes. While allergies or environmental conditions may cause your eyes to burn at various times, the symptom is often due to a lack of vitamins A and B_2. Vitamin A is responsible for tissue repair and also helps the body resist infection. B_2 regulates cell respiration. Together, these vitamins keep the eye cells strong and moist.

Dosage: You need 5,000 IU of vitamin A per day and 1.3–1.7 mg of vitamin B_2.

Food Sources: The best sources of vitamin A include green and yellow fruits and vegetables (spinach and raw carrots, e.g.). Vitamin B_2 is found in blackstrap molasses, nuts, organ meats, whole grains, and brewer's yeast.

Kidney Dysfunction

Description: Very simply, this condition refers to improper functioning of the kidney. It can occur as a result of some sort of trauma or injury, but it is most likely the result of a deficiency of pantothenic acid. This vitamin aids in the digestive process, converting food into available energy. When digestion is working properly the liquid waste products are excreted by the kidneys in a normal manner.

Dosage: You need between .5 and 10 mg of pantothenic acid per day.

Food Sources: It is found in brewer's yeast, legumes, organ meats, salmon, wheat germ, whole grains, and fresh orange juice.

Kidney Stones

Description: Kidney stones are rocklike substances formed in the urinary tract from the mineral salts in the urine. The stones vary in size from grains of sand to actual stones that occupy much space in the kidney. Although the cause is often unknown, medical treatment involves large amounts of water, a special diet, and medication. It is also possible that kidney stones form due to a lack of vitamin B_6 and magnesium. Vitamin B_6 controls the production of oxalic acid, which is that part of the urine that binds together to form a stone. Magnesium makes the urine more solvent so the stones cannot form.

Dosage: You need 1.8-2.2 mg of vitamin B_6 and 300-350 mg of magnesium daily.

Food Sources: Vitamin B_6 comes from blackstrap molasses, brewer's yeast, green leafy vegetables, meat, organ meats, wheat germ, whole grains, prunes, brown rice, and peas. Magnesium is supplied by bran, honey, green vegetables (including spinach), nuts, seafood, bone meal, kelp tablets, and bran flakes.

Lesions

Description: A lesion is an abnormal change in a body part or an organ due to an injury or a disease. When a lesion occurs on the lips, mouth, eyes, skin, or genitals it is often due to a deficiency of vitamin B_2. This vitamin specifically protects the body through antibody formation, cell respiration, and metabolism regulation. These three basic functions increase the strength and resistance of the body to injury or illness.

Dosage: Vitamin B_2 should be taken in 1.3–1.7 mg doses per day.

Food Sources: Vitamin B_2 is found in blackstrap molasses, nuts, organ meats, whole grains, and brewer's yeast.

Liver Dysfunction (Fat Intolerance)

Description: This is the inability of the liver to metabolize fat. The result can be excessive weight gain or secondary contributions to heart disease. Proper functioning can be restored through adequate intake of choline. Choline is directly responsible for regulating the activity of the liver, producing lecithin (an emulsifier), and metabolizing fats and cholesterol.

Dosage: There is no specific recommendation for the daily intake of choline.

Food Sources: Choline is found in brewer's yeast, fish, legumes, organ meats, soybeans, wheat germ, egg yolks, lecithin, and peanuts.

Loss of Smell

Description: This is a result of temporary or permanent destruction of the olfactory sense. While physical trauma may cause the disorder, a lack of vitamin A can also be responsible. Vitamin A is involved with tissue repair, which provides new and healthy cells throughout the olfactory sense system.

Dosage: You need 5,000 IU of vitamin A per day.

Food Sources: It is found in green and yellow fruits and vegetables (spinach and raw carrots, e.g.), milk, fish liver oil, and beef liver.

Memory Lapses

Description: Faulty memory is most often due to poor learning of the material in question. Memory loss can also occur because of a nutritional deficiency of the B complex vitamins and iron. The B complex vitamins help keep the nervous system functioning properly and subsequently improve learning capacity. This leads to better retention and memory. Iron promotes hemoglobin production for healthier red blood cells. These cells carry oxygen to the brain cells for increased nourishment. Then brain cells function more efficiently to promote an improved memory.

Dosage: There are individual doses for each of the B complex vitamins (see the chart in the appendix). You also need 10–18 mg of iron a day.

Food Sources: The best sources of the B complex vitamins include blackstrap molasses, brewer's yeast, liver, wheat germ, and whole grains. Iron is found in blackstrap molasses, eggs, fish, organ meats, poultry, and wheat germ.

Memory Loss

Description: The inability to remember names, faces, dates, etc., is often due to the aging process—or so we think. Actually, a poor memory is usually the result of a diminished learning capacity. This problem can have several causes, such as communication barriers, improper memorization techniques, and a deficiency of vitamin B_1. This vitamin helps regulate the functions of the nervous system with specific reference to a person's ability to learn. Material that is learned better is retained better, and there is no appreciable memory loss.

Dosage: You need 1-1.5 mg of vitamin B_1 daily.

Food Sources: Vitamin B_1 is found in blackstrap molasses, brewer's yeast, brown rice, fish, meats, nuts, organ meats, poultry, and wheat germ.

Ménière's Syndrome

Description: This is a disease of the inner ear that usually involves a single ear and is most common in men over age 40. The syndrome is caused by a blow to the ear, an infection, an allergic reaction, a congenital condition, or other unknown factors. Ménière's syndrome is characterized by dizziness, nausea, and vomiting. There may also be a ringing in the ear accompanied by headaches, a disturbed sense of balance, and a loss of hearing. While a vitamin deficiency has not been suggested as a cause, niacin has been shown to be an effective treatment. Niacin serves several functions specific to alleviating Ménière's syndrome. The vitamin helps regulate the nervous system, improve circulation, and control metabolic processes, all of which combine to relieve the symptoms of this condition.

Dosage: You should have 10-18 mg of niacin daily.

Food Sources: Niacin is found in brewer's yeast, seafood, lean meats, milk, poultry, dessicated liver, rhubarb, and peanuts.

Menopausal Symptoms

Description: *Menopause* refers to the period in life when menstruation becomes irregular and eventually ceases. Hormonal imbalance occurs and is usually accompanied by some psychological and behavioral changes. Menopause usually occurs in women between the ages of 45 and 55. If it occurs prematurely, menopause may be due to a vitamin deficiency, especially of vitamins D and E. Both vitamins help maintain a healthy nervous system, and vitamin E improves circulation. These combined functions can prevent hormonal changes and reduce the incidence of premature menopausal symptoms.

Dosage: You need 400 IU of vitamin D and 12–15 IU of vitamin E daily.

Food Sources: Vitamin D is found in egg yolks, organ meats, bone meal, sunlight, milk, salmon, and tuna fish. Vitamin E comes from dark green vegetables, eggs, liver, organ meats, wheat germ, vegetable oils, oatmeal, peanuts, and tomatoes.

Menstrual Cramps

Description: While there is no evidence that menstrual cramps are caused by nutritional deficiencies, it is possible to ease them or even relieve them with adequate consumption of vitamin B complex and calcium. The B complex vitamins help maintain the healthy functioning of the nervous system, and calcium regulates nerve transmission and muscle contraction. Together, these nutrients may be able to ease the intensity of the cramps.

Dosage: Each vitamin in the B complex has its own specific dosage (see the chart in the appendix). You need 800–1,400 mg of calcium a day.

Food Sources: The basic sources of the B complex vitamins include blackstrap molasses, brewer's yeast, liver, wheat germ, and whole grains. Calcium comes from milk, cheese, molasses, yogurt, bone meal, dolomite, and almonds.

Mental Illness

Description: *Mental illness* refers to a category of diseases of the mind. These include emotional instability, a general inability to deal with the rigors of daily living, and more severe conditions such as schizophrenia and depression. The causes of these illnesses are many, and they are best treated with professional help. However, it is becoming increasingly clear to these professionals that mental illness may be related to a nutritional deficiency of B complex vitamins. More specifically, niacin has been used in treatment. Niacin has a direct, facilitative effect on circulation and metabolism. This leads to more efficient functioning of the brain cells, resulting in an improvement of an individual's mental condition.

Dosage: You need 13–18 mg of niacin a day.

Food Sources: Niacin comes from brewer's yeast, seafood, lean meats, milk, poultry, dessicated liver, rhubarb, and peanuts.

Miscarriage

Description: This is an abrupt termination of pregnancy due to expulsion of the fetus, usually between the fourth month and the due date. Many things can cause a miscarriage, especially physical trauma and sometimes emotional stress. However, it is sometimes possible to prevent a miscarriage with adequate supplies of vitamins E and K. Both these vitamins are involved in circulatory regulation, which will provide nourishment for the fetus, the placenta, and the uterus.

Dosage: You need 12–15 IU of vitamin E a day. There is no specific recommendation for the daily intake of vitamin K.

Food Sources: Vitamin E is found in dark green vegetables, eggs, liver, wheat germ, vegetable oils, oatmeal, peanuts, and tomatoes. Vitamin K comes from green leafy vegetables, safflower oil, blackstrap molasses, yogurt, oatmeal, and beef liver.

Muscle Cramps

Description: A cramp is an extreme and sustained contraction of a muscle, without relaxation, caused by constant firing of the nerve cells. Overexertion and fatigue can lead to muscle cramps, but the most likely cause is a lack of potassium. Potassium is responsible for regulating muscle contractions and calming the nervous system. Additionally, a deficiency in pantothenic acid and calcium can lead to the occurrence of cramps. Pantothenic acid is involved with energy conversion, so the muscles can be nourished and worked properly. Calcium regulates muscle contraction and nerve transmission and tranquilization, similar to potassium. The combination of these three nutrients serves to reduce the incidence and severity of muscle cramps.

Dosage: While there is no recommended dosage for potassium, you need .5-10 mg of pantothenic acid and 800-1,400 mg of calcium daily.

Food Sources: Pantothenic acid comes from brewer's yeast, legumes, organ meats, salmon, wheat germ, whole grains, and fresh orange juice. Potassium is found in dates, figs, green peppers, peaches, tomato juice, blackstrap molasses, peanuts, raisins, seafood, bananas, potatoes, and sunflower seeds. Calcium is provided by milk, cheese, molasses, yogurt, bone meal, dolomite, almonds, and beef liver.

Muscle Spasms

Description: A spasm, or twitch, is a sudden, involuntary contraction of a muscle or muscle group that may be accompanied by pain. The contraction may be caused by a disturbance in circulation, a neurological problem, a disease, or a nutritional deficiency. A lack of vitamin D, calcium, phosphorus, sodium, or potassium can create spasmodic reactions. All these nutrients help regulate and control muscle activity and maintain a tranquilizing effect on the nervous system.

Dosage: You need 400 IU of vitamin D, 800-1,400 mg of calcium, and 800 mg of phosphorus a day. There are no specific dosages for either sodium or potassium, but an intake of 100-300 mg daily has been suggested for both.

Food Sources: Vitamin D is found in egg yolks, organ meats, bone meal, sunlight, milk, salmon, and tuna fish. Calcium comes from milk, cheese, molasses, yogurt, bone meal, dolomite, almonds, and beef liver. Phosphorus is supplied by eggs, fish, grains, glandular meats, meat, poultry, milk, and yogurt. You get sodium from salt, milk, cheese, and seafood. Potassium is found in dates, figs, peaches, tomato juice, blackstrap molasses, peanuts, raisins, seafood, apricots, bananas, potatoes, and green pepers.

Muscular Pain

Description: This can be acute or chronic pain within a muscle caused by a blow to the area, overexertion, a strain, or a tear. The pain is amplified by a lack of biotin in the system. Biotin promotes cell growth, and new cells ease the pain caused by the trauma to the old cells.

Dosage: You should have 150–300 mcg of biotin daily.

Food Sources: You get biotin in legumes, whole grains, organ meats, brewer's yeast, and egg yolks.

Myopia

Description: This is a defect in vision resulting in extreme nearsightedness. It may be caused by a lack of vitamin D, which is responsible for the maintenance of nervous system activity. Although the relationship is somewhat unclear at this time, it is hypothesized that improved nervous system activity may lead to improved vision.

Dosage: You need 400 IU of vitamin D daily.

Food Sources: Vitamin D occurs naturally in egg yolks, organ meats, bone meal, sunlight, milk, salmon, and tuna fish.

Nausea

Description: This unpleasant sensation in the pit of the stomach is often a warning that vomiting may soon occur. Nausea results from a disagreement between foods we eat and our digestive systems. The nausea is further enhanced by a lack of niacin. Niacin aids circulation in the body, hydrochloric acid production, and metabolism. All these functions aid digestion, thereby decreasing nausea.

Dosage: You need 13–18 mg of niacin daily.

Food Sources; Niacin is found in brewer's yeast, seafood, lean meats, milk, poultry, dessicated liver, and peanuts.

Nerve Degeneration

Description: This condition occurs when the nerves begin to degenerate or even disintegrate. Obviously, a loss of neurological functioning accompanies this problem. While certain cases of nerve degeneration are caused by physical trauma, other cases may be due to a deficiency of vitamin B_{12}. This vitamin is involved in the synthesis of DNA and RNA and in the maintenance of the nerve-cell membranes. A deficiency causes a deterioration of these membranes and the subsequent degeneration of the nerve itself.

Dosage: You need 3 mcg of vitamin B_{12} a day.

Food Sources: Vitamin B_{12} is found in cheese, fish, milk, organ meats, and eggs.

Nervous Tension

Description: This is just a feeling of uneasiness, such as being uptight or under too much pressure. Stress is the main cause of nervous tension, but emotions such as anxiety, frustration, and anger can also create the condition. A lack of vitamin B complex and vitamin C has also been implicated as a possible cause. While taking these vitamins may not prevent nervous tension, it should decrease the intensity of the reaction. Additionally, taking vitamin B complex and vitamin C will improve the functional efficiency of the nervous system, which will also decrease the stress response.

Dosage: The B complex vitamins each have individual doses (see the chart in the appendix). You need 60 mg of vitamin C daily.

Food Sources: The B complex vitamins are generally supplied by blackstrap molasses, brewer's yeast, liver, wheat germ, and whole grains. Vitamin C is supplied by citrus fruits, cantaloupes, broccoli, green peppers, and potatoes.

Nervousness

Description: A person who is nervous appears to be anxious, excitable, tense, edgy, and so on. Usually, the nervousness is caused by some sort of stress or uncertainty. However, it is very likely that the nervousness is caused by nutrient deficiencies. The vitamins and minerals whose lack contributes to this condition are B_1, B_{12}, niacin, pangamic acid, D, calcium, magnesium, phosphorus, and potassium. All these nutrients are involved in the regulation of the nervous system, through maintenance of structure, control of transmission rates, or tranquilization of the entire system. Additionally, vitamin D, calcium, phosphorus, and potassium exert control of heart rate and rhythm. Since the heart speeds up when you are nervous it is logical that, if the rate can be controlled, nervousness will subside or possibly not occur.

Dosage: Only pangamic acid and potassium do not have a recommended daily dosage. You should receive 1–1.5 mg of B_1, 3 mcg of B_{12}, 13–18 mg of niacin, 400 IU of D, 800–1,400 mg of calcium, 300–350 mg of magnesium, and 800 mg of phosphorus.

Food Sources:

B_1: Blackstrap molasses, brewer's yeast, brown rice, fish, meat, nuts, organ meats, poultry, wheat germ.

B_{12}: Cheese, fish, milk, organ meats, cottage cheese, beef liver, tuna fish, eggs.

Niacin: Brewer's yeast, seafood, lean meats, milk, poultry, dessicated liver, cooked rhubarb, chicken, peanuts.

Pangamic Acid: Brewer's yeast, brown rice, rare meat, seeds, whole grains, organ meats.

D: Egg yolks, organ meats, bone meal, sunlight, beef liver, milk, salmon, tuna.

Calcium: Milk, cheese, molasses, yogurt, bone meal, dolomite, almonds, beef liver.

Magnesium: Bran, honey, green vegetables (spinach, etc.), nuts, seafood, bone meal, kelp tablets.

Phosphorus: Eggs, fish, grains, glandular meats, meat, poultry, yellow cheese, calf liver, milk, yogurt.

Potassium: Dates, figs, peaches, tomato juice, blackstrap molasses, peanuts, raisins, seafood, dried apricots, bananas, baked flounder, baked potato, sunflower seeds.

Night Blindness

Description: The absence of vision in the dark, or an inability to see clearly in the dark, is caused by a lack of vitamin A. This vitamin serves specifically to improve night vision.

Dosage: You should have 5,000 IU of vitamin A daily.

Food Sources: Vitamin A is found in green and yellow fruits and vegetables (spinach and raw carrots, etc.), milk, fish liver oil, and beef liver.

Nosebleeds

Description: Hemorrhaging (bleeding) from the nose is caused by physical trauma or a lack of vitamins C and K. Vitamin C aids the healing process and vitamin K enhances the blood-clotting ability of the body.

Dosage: You require 60 mg of vitamin C daily. There is no specific recommendation for vitamin K.

Food Sources: You get vitamin C from citrus fruits, cantaloupe, green peppers, broccoli, and potatoes. Vitamin K is found in green leafy vegetables, safflower oil, blackstrap molasses, yogurt, oatmeal, and beef liver.

Numbness (Limbs)

Description: Numbness is a lack of feeling or sensation in a body part. Most often numbness occurs in the hands, fingers, feet, and toes. The lack of feeling is usually due to poor circulation in that area. A deficiency of vitamin B_1 and calcium can be the cause of the circulatory problem and resultant numbness. Vitamin B_1 helps regulate circulation, and calcium controls heart rhythm and thus the flow of blood throughout the body.

Dosage: You require 1–1.5 mg of vitamin B_1 and 800–1,400 mg of calcium a day.

Food Sources: Vitamin B_1 is found in blackstrap molasses, brewer's yeast, brown rice, fish, meats, nuts, organ meats, poultry, and wheat germ. Calcium comes from milk, cheese, molasses, yogurt, bone meal, dolomite, almonds, and beef liver.

Obesity

Description: Many people feel that the number one health problem in this country is obesity. Obesity is a condition in which there is an abnormally excessive amount of fat on the body. Usually, a person is considered obese if his or her weight is 30 percent above the average weight for the individual's age, gender, and height.

The two most prevalent causes of obesity are inactivity and overeating. Additionally, obesity may be caused by a nutritional deficiency of iodine and phosphorus. Both of these minerals are involved in regulating metabolism and energy production. Since obesity is a result of an energy imbalance, where the energy (food) taken in is greater than the energy expended, it is easy to see how these minerals may help overcome the problem.

Dosage: You should have 150 mcg of iodine and 800 mg of phosphorus daily.

Food Sources: Iodine comes from seafood, kelp tablets, and salt. Phosphorus is found in eggs, fish, grains, meat, poultry, yellow cheese, calf liver, milk, and yogurt.

Osteomalacia (Softening of the Bones)

Description: This is an abnormal bone condition in adults, similar to rickets in children, in which the bones gradually soften due to a deficiency of vitamin D, calcium, and phosphorus. These nutrients are directly responsible for the formation and growth of healthy bones, and a lack of these substances will lead to osteomalacia. The condition can also be caused by an abnormality in the manner in which the body uses these substances. Prompt treatment with vitamins and minerals can cure the problem.

Dosage: You need 400 IU of vitamin D, 800–1,400 mg of calcium, and 800 mg of phosphorus daily.

Food Sources: Vitamin D comes from egg yolks, organ meats, bone meal, sunlight, milk, salmon, and tuna fish. Calcium is found in milk, cheese, molasses, yogurt, bone meal, dolomite, almonds, and beef liver. Phosphorus is supplied by eggs, fish, grains, glandular meats, meat, poultry, yellow cheese, milk, and yogurt.

Osteoporosis

Description: Osteoporosis has been called "brittle bones," but it is more accurately a thinning of the bone due to insufficient deposits of calcium. A lack of vitamin D also contributes to osteoporosis because vitamin D promotes calcium absorption. This bone-softening process usually occurs in women after middle age. That is why it is so difficult for a broken bone to heal in an elderly person. Both calcium and vitamin D aid in the growth and development of strong bones.

Dosage: You need 800–1,400 mg of calcium a day, as well as 400 IU of vitamin D.

Food Sources: Calcium is found in milk, cheese, molasses, yogurt, bone meal, dolomite, almonds, and beef liver. Vitamin D comes from egg yolks, organ meats, bone meal, sunlight, beef liver, milk, salmon, and tuna fish.

Pellagra

Description: This condition is a result of a niacin deficiency, and its symptoms include skin rashes (dermatitis), dementia, and diarrhea, and, in severe cases, death. Although the disease is rare in North American, incidences have been reported among alcoholics, diabetics, cancer victims, and sufferers of chronic diarrhea. Perhaps these conditions hamper the body's ability to absorb and utilize niacin. Niacin's main functions in the prevention of pellagra include promotion of circulation and metabolism, which seem to nourish and strengthen the cells.

Dosage: You need 13–18 mg of niacin daily.

Food Sources: Niacin is found in brewer's yeast, seafood, lean meats, milk, poultry, dessicated liver, and peanuts.

Phlebitis

Description: Phlebitis is the inflammation of a vein. It is usually associated with thrombosis, which is a blood clot in the vein. Phlebitis is common in the legs, and it may occur in people who are overweight or who have circulatory problems, such as varicose veins. The area surrounding the phlebitis becomes red and painful. The cause of the condition is often unknown. A lack of vitamin E may not be responsible for phlebitis, but adequate amounts of the vitamin can provide relief. That is because vitamin E helps improve circulation throughout the body.

Dosage: You need 12–15 IU of vitamin E daily.

Food Sources: Vitamin E is supplied by dark green vegetables, eggs, liver, organ meats, wheat ferm, vegetable oils, oatmeal, peanuts, and tomatoes.

Premature Aging

Description: The early onset of signs and symptoms of aging is usually due to excessive stress or trauma. However, the graying hair, the arthritic hands, or the loss of motor control can also be due to a deficiency of pantothenic acid. This nutrient helps regulate the energy conversion process and the growth of new cells. Both of these functions tend to keep the body and its systems young.

Dosage: You need .5–10 mg of pantothenic acid a day.

Food Sources: Pantothenic acid is found in brewer's yeast, legumes, organ meats, salmon, wheat germ, whole grains, and fresh orange juice.

Prickly Heat

Description: Prickly heat is an itchy rash made up of minute reddish pimples. It usually occurs in summertime due to excessive sweating and chafing. While vitamin C deficiency is not a cause of this condition, the nutrient is used in its treatment. Vitamin C promotes the healing processes of the body as well as increases the body's resistance to external infections. Prickly heat is not an infection, per se, but the body responds as if it were. That is why vitamin C is effective as a treatment.

Dosage: You need 60 mg of vitamin C a day.

Food Sources: Vitamin C is supplied by citrus fruits, cantaloupe, broccoli, green peppers, and potatoes.

Psoriasis

Description: Psoriasis is a skin disease characterized by itchy red patches that become covered with loose silvery patches. The eruptions can appear all over the body, but usually occur on the scalp, forearms, elbows, knees, and legs. The condition tends to run in families. Although the cause is unknown, psoriasis seems to be related to a deficiency of vitamins A and F. Vitamin A is responsible for maintaining healthy cells, and vitamin F promotes vital organ respiration. Together, these nutrients work to keep the skin from being susceptible to psoriasis.

Dosage: You need 5,000 IU of vitamin A daily. Also, 10 percent of your daily calories should contain vitamin F (unsaturated fatty acids).

Food Sources: Vitamin A comes from green and yellow fruits and vegetables (apricots, spinach, and raw carrots, e.g.), and beef liver. Vitamin F (unsaturated fatty acids) should comprise 10 percent of your total daily caloric intake.

Pyorrhea

Description: This is a disease of the mouth in which the gum tissue gradually separates from the tooth and a pocket of pus forms between the soft gum tissues and the hard tooth surface. As bacteria, food debris, and saliva collect in the pockets the destructive process is intensified. The bone adjacent to the infected area disappears, more attaching tissue is lost, and the pocket deepens and widens. The tooth eventually loosens to create further irritation.

While nutritional deficiencies may not always cause pyorrhea, adequate amounts of vitamins C and D and calcium and phosphorus should prevent the disease from occurring. Vitamins C and D both promote healthy tooth formation. Calcium and phosphorus are also responsible for creating healthy teeth and gums. It is imperative, in this case, that these nutrients be ingested in the proper amounts.

Dosage: You need 60 mg of vitamin C, 400 IU of vitamin D, 800–1,400 mg of calcium, and 800 mg of phosphorus daily.

Food Sources: Vitamin C comes from citrus fruits, cantaloupe, broccoli, green peppers, and potatoes. Vitamin D is found in egg yolks, organ meats, bone meal, sunlight, milk, salmon, and tuna fish. Calcium is supplied by milk, cheese, molasses, yogurt, bone meal, dolomite, almonds, and beef liver. Phosphorus comes from eggs, fish, grains, glandular meats, meat, poultry, yellow cheese, milk, and yogurt.

Red, Sore Tongue

Description: The inflammation and painful feeling of the tongue is due to a lack of vitamin B_2. This vitamin regulates cell respiration and metabolism, both of which serve integral functions in the healing process.

Dosage: You should have 1.3–1.7 mg of vitamin B_2 daily.

Food Sources: Vitamin B_2 comes from blackstrap molasses, nuts, organ meats, whole grains, Brussels sprouts, and brewer's yeast.

Respiratory Failure

Description: Problems with, or even a complete cessation of breathing is rarely considered the result of a nutritional deficiency. However, a lack of the vitamin B complex and potassium may have a contributory effect. The B complex vitamins maintain a healthy and effective nervous system. Potassium also controls the activity of the nervous system as well as the process of muscle contraction. Thus, these two nutrients can influence the activity of the breathing muscles. It should also be remembered that respiratory failure often accompanies cardiac arrest, and that is why similar nutrients are involved.

Dosage: The B complex vitamins each have individual requirements (see the chart in the appendix). There is no specific daily dosage for potassium, but it is suggested that you have 100–300 mg a day.

Food Sources: The basic sources of the B complex vitamins include blackstrap molasses, brewer's yeast, liver, wheat germ, and whole grains. Potassium is supplied by dates, figs, peaches, tomato juice, blackstrap molasses, peanuts, raisins, seafood, apricots, bananas, potatoes, and green peppers.

Restlessness

Description: The general feeling of uneasiness, or just being fidgety, is characteristic of restlessness. While emotional pressures or lack of sleep may create this feeling, it is often due to a deficiency of pantothenic acid. This nutrient aids in energy metabolism and the body's ability to use other vitamins, thereby regulating many of the physiological processes. One of the results is a feeling of calmness.

Dosage: You should have .5-10 mg of pantothenic acid a day.

Food Sources: Pantothenic acid is found in brewer's yeast, legumes, organ meats, salmon, wheat germ, whole grains, and fresh orange juice.

Rheumatism

Description: Rheumatism is a painful disorder involving the joints and bones and the tissues supporting them. The condition is very similar to arthritis in that the joints and tissues can become inflamed, thus causing pain. Wear and tear on the bones due to aging is often cited as a major cause. Stress can also lead to rheumatism. Additionally, a nutritional deficiency of vitamins B_6, C, and D and calcium may create this disorder. Vitamin B_6 aids the pain of rheumatism by improving the functioning of the nervous system and increasing the body's resistance to stress. Vitamin C regulates the production of collagen, which is the support tissue of bones. All these functions combine to reduce the incidence of rheumatism.

Dosage: You need 1.8-2.2 mg of vitamin B_6, 60 mg of vitamin C, 400 IU of vitamin D, and 800-1,400 mg of calcium a day.

Food Sources: Vitamin B_6 comes from blackstrap molasses, brewer's yeast, green leafy vegetables, meat, organ meats, wheat germ, whole grains, prunes, brown rice, and peas. Vitamin C is supplied by citrus fruits, cantaloupe, broccoli, green peppers, and potatoes. Vitamin D is found in egg yolks, organ meats, bone meal, sunlight, milk, salmon, and tuna fish. Calcium occurs in milk, cheese, molasses, yogurt, bone meal, dolomite, almonds, and beef liver.

Rickets

Description: Rickets is a bone disorder of children that results in malformations, retarded or distorted growth, and soft bones. This is due solely to a lack of vitamin D. The main function of vitamin D is to promote bone growth by increasing the body's ability to absorb calcium and phosphorus, which are the two minerals responsible for proper bone development.

Dosage: You need 400 IU of vitamin D a day.

Food Sources: Vitamin D is found in egg yolks, organ meats, bone meal, milk, and sunlight.

Rough/Bumpy Skin (Also see Rough/Dry Skin)

Description: This condition occurs due to a hardening of the hair follicles along with some other skin changes. It used to be called "toad skin," but the medical term is *follicular hyperkeratosis*. It looks like goose pimples, but the lumps do not go away. The problem is caused by a deficiency of vitamin A, whose primary function in this case is body tissue (skin) reparation and maintenance. Since vitamin A deficiency also causes dry skin, the two conditions may occur simultaneously.

Dosage: A daily dose of 5,000 IU of vitamin A is required.

Food Sources: Vitamin A comes from green and yellow fruits and vegetables (apricots, spinach, and raw carrots, e.g.), milk, fish liver oil, and beef liver.

Rough/Dry Skin
(Also see Rough/Bumpy Skin)

Description: Hardened skin lacks the appropriate oils and moisture. While dry skin often occurs due to wind, rain, or cold, it can also result from a nutrient deficiency. The specific nutrients involved are vitamin A, which aids in tissue repair; vitamin B complex, which regulates metabolic and energy production processes; vitamin F, which promotes glandular activity (*read* oil production) and vital organ respiration (*read* moisture production); and potassium, which helps regulate cell growth. All these nutrients facilitate the growth of new and healthy skin cells.

Dosage: You need 5,000 IU of vitamin A per day. The specific amount of the B complex vitamins varies with each vitamin (see appendix). Vitamin F should comprise 10 percent of your total daily calories, and potassium intake, though there is no specific recommended daily dosage, should be 100–300 mg daily.

Food Sources: Vitamin A is found in green and yellow fruits and vegetables (spinach and raw carrots, e.g.), milk, fish liver oil, and beef liver. The B complex vitamins come from brewer's yeast, liver, blackstrap molasses, and whole grains. Vitamin F is found in vegetable oils, wheat germ, and sunflower seeds. Potassium occurs in dates, figs, peaches, tomato juice, blackstrap molasses, peanuts, raisins, seafood, bananas, potato, sunflower seeds, and green peppers.

Schizophrenia

Description: Schizophrenia is a serious mental disorder characterized by irrational thinking, disturbed emotions, and a breakdown in communication with others. Schizophrenia is a form of psychosis. Although the cause is virtually unknown, a biochemical breakdown along with negative personal experiences has been suggested. Nutritional deficiencies may not be related to the occurrence of this disorder, but psychotherapists have found some treatment success with nutritional supplementation. Specifically, adequate doses, and sometimes megadoses, of the vitamin B complex and vitamins C and E have proven effective. These vitamins combine to regulate both the nervous system and the circulatory system. The result is more effective brain function. However, vitamin therapy for schizophrenia should be undertaken only while in professional care.

Dosage: The B complex vitamins each have their individual doses, and these are provided in the chart in the appendix. You need 60 mg of vitamin C and 12–15 IU of vitamin E daily.

Food Sources: The basic sources of the B complex vitamins include blackstrap molasses, brewer's yeast, liver, wheat germ, and whole grains. Vitamin C is supplied by citrus fruits, cantaloupe, broccoli, green peppers, and potatoes. Vitamin E is found in dark green vegetables, eggs, liver, organ meats, wheat germ, vegetable oils, oatmeal, peanuts, and tomatoes.

Shingles
(Herpes Zoster)

Description: Shingles is a condition characterized by an inflammation along the course of the sensory nerve that comes out from the spine. The disorder is also accompanied by corps of small blisters and great pain. The nerves that are affected are usually those on the abdomen and chest, and only on one side of the body. Shingles is caused by the same virus that causes chicken pox. Susceptibility to shingles is increased when there is a deficiency of vitamin B_{12}. This vitamin is responsible for keeping cells alive and the nervous system healthy. A strong nervous system would decrease the possibility of getting shingles.

Dosage: You need 3 mcg of vitamin B_{12} a day.

Food Sources: Vitamin B_{12} is found in cheese, fish, milk, organ meats, and eggs.

Shortness of Breath

Description: Shortness of breath occurs when a person is unable to breathe normally or unable to catch his or her breath. Exercise, emotional or physical trauma, and illness can cause shortness of breath. It can also come from a lack of vitamin B_1. Vitamin B_1 regulates many bodily processes, but those that will dissipate this symptom include metabolism and energy conversion, circulation, and nervous system maintenance. Together, these functions will help the body begin operating normally, which includes appropriate respiration.

Dosage: You should have 1–1.5 mg of vitamin B_1 a day.

Food Sources: Vitamin B_1 occurs in blackstrap molasses, brewer's yeast, brown rice, fish, meat, nuts, organ meats, poultry, and wheat germ.

Sinus Trouble

Description: The symptoms of sinus trouble include a runny nose, a stuffy head, an inability to breathe, and a headache. They are due to an inflammation or congestion of the canals (sinuses) that surround the eyes and nose. Antihistamines tend to relieve the problem temporarily, but since a lack of vitamin A can also cause sinus trouble, it may make more sense to alleviate the symptom through proper nutrition. It is the tissue repair function of vitamin A that reduces the inflammation and resolves sinusitis.

Dosage: You need 5,000 IU of vitamin A daily.

Food Sources: Vitamin A is found in green and yellow fruits and vegetables (spinach and raw carrots, e.g.), milk, fish liver oil, and beef liver.

Skin Pallor

Description: A loss of color in the skin, which results in a pale or grayish appearance, is often due to an iron deficiency. Iron is necessary for the production of hemoglobin, which carries oxygen and gives red blood cells their color. Without enough iron, and subsequently enough hemoglobin, skin cells will become undernourished and lose their color. A similar effect occurs when circulation to a body part is decreased. The skin becomes pale, gray, and sometimes even bluish.

Dosage: You need 10–18 mg of iron per day.

Food Sources: Iron comes from blackstrap molasses, eggs, fish, organ meats, poultry, and wheat germ.

Skin Sores

Description: Skin sores are characterized by inflammation, redness, and scabs on the skin. While the cause of the sores may vary, they are often due to a deficiency of copper. This mineral regulates both the healing processes of the body and the formation of red blood cells. Together these functions can overcome this condition.

Dosage: You need 2 mg of copper a day.

Food Sources: Copper is found in legumes, nuts, organ meats, seafood, raisins, molasses, and bone meal.

Soft Tooth Enamel

Description: The weakness or softness in the outer protective layer of the tooth is usually due to a nutritional deficiency of vitamins A and D and calcium. Vitamin A serves a secondary function in strengthening the tooth enamel through its role in tissue repair. Vitamin D and calcium are both directly responsible for the formation of strong bones and teeth.

Dosage: You require 5,000 IU of vitamin A, 400 IU of vitamin D, and 800–1,400 mg of calcium a day.

Food Sources: Vitamin A is found in green and yellow fruits and vegetables (spinach and raw carrots, e.g.), milk, fish liver oil, and beef liver. Vitamin D comes from egg yolks, organ meats, bone meal, sunlight, beef liver, milk, salmon, and tuna fish. Calcium occurs in milk, cheese, molasses, yogurt, bone meal, dolomite, almonds, and beef liver.

Sore Throat
(Pharyngitis, Tonsillitis)

Description: A sore throat is an inflammation and soreness of any part of or all of the throat area. It can be caused by an infection, air pollution, smoking, or misusing the voice. A sore throat is usually a sign that a more acute infection will follow. Adequate daily doses of vitamin C, which helps prevent infection in general, may prevent a sore throat from occurring. Once you have a sore throat, vitamin C may be able to speed up the healing process. However, there are no guarantees that the condition will not return.

Dosage: You should have 60 mg of vitamin C daily.

Food Sources: Vitamin C is supplied by citrus fruits, cantaloupe, green peppers, broccoli, and potatoes.

Sterility

Description: Sterility is the inability of a female to become pregnant or the inability of a male to impregnate a female. The cause is usually genetic, but it can also be the result of a nutritional deficiency. Vitamin E and zinc are the two most important nutrients implicated in this problem. Vitamin E promotes fertility and male potency. Zinc helps regulate reproductive organ growth and development in males and females. Together, these nutrients may alleviate the problem.

Dosage: Between 12 and 15 IU of vitamin E is required daily, along with 15 mg of zinc.

Food Sources: You get vitamin E from dark green vegetables, eggs, liver, organ meats, wheat germ, vegetable oils, oatmeal, peanuts, and tomatoes. Zinc is found in brewer's yeast, liver, seafood, soybeans, spinach, sunflower seeds, and mushrooms.

Stress

Description: Stress refers to any situation we perceive as demanding and that requires us to make adjustments in our behavior or thought patterns. Put simply, stress is a condition of severe strain or pressure. The cause of stress can be emotional, physical, and even nutritional. Poor dietary habits leading to inadequate vitamin and mineral intake increase susceptibility to stress. It is necessary to receive an adequate daily supply of every vitamin and mineral, but the two most popular stress vitamins are B complex and C. Remember, all the nutrients are important to combat stress and to prevent it from affecting us in a debilitating manner.

Dosage: Try to get the recommended daily dosages of each vitamin and mineral. (See appendix.)

Food Sources: A well-balanced, nutritionally sound diet will provide all the vitamins and minerals you need to manage stress effectively.

Sunburn

Description: Sunburn damages the skin and can even cause second-degree burns. Severe sunburn covers the skin with large, watery blisters and makes it sensitive to the touch. The danger of infection always exists when blisters are present. Furthermore, if the sunburn covers a large area of the body, shock can result. When the skin starts to heal there may be scars and unsightly patches. The best preventive measure for sunburn is to stay out of the sun. For those who must be in the sun, lotions are made that contain para-aminobenzoic acid (PABA). PABA is a sunscreen that prevents you from burning. If you do get a burn, external application of PABA can speed the healing process.

Dosage: There is no specific requirement for PABA, but 10–100 mg has been suggested as a daily dose.

Food Sources: PABA is found in blackstrap molasses, brewer's yeast, liver, organ meats, and wheat germ.

Susceptibility to Infections

Description: Fatigue, overexertion, or a previous illness can tend to lower your resistance. A lack of vitamins A and C can also hinder the ability of the immune system to protect the body. Both vitamins strengthen the immune system and increase the body's ability to resist infection.

Dosage: You need 5,000 IU of vitamin A and 60 mg of vitamin C a day.

Food Sources: Vitmain A is found in green and yellow fruits and vegetables (spinach and raw carrots, e.g.), fish liver oil, and beef liver. You get vitamin C from citrus fruits, cantaloupe, green peppers, broccoli, and potatoes.

Tetany

Description: Tetany is a condition of intermittent tonic muscle contractions, often accompanied by pain. The most characteristic signs of this disorder are the inward muscular spasms of the wrist (Trousseau's sign) and lockjaw. Tetany is caused by an abnormal metabolism of calcium, which results in lowered blood calcium levels. This affects the body's ability to control the rate and intensity of muscular contractions. Hence, tetany can occur.

Dosage: You need 800–1,400 mg of calcium daily.

Food Sources: Calcium is found in milk, cheese, molasses, yogurt, bone meal, dolomite, almonds, and beef liver.

Tremors

Description: A tremor is a shaking of a body part due to overexcitability of a muscle. Nervous system damage due to physical trauma can lead to this condition. Also, a lack of magnesium can cause tremors. Magnesium is a catalyst in the body's utilization of the macronutrients (carbohydrates, proteins, and fats) as well as calcium, phosphorus, and possibly potassium. These last three minerals are involved in the regulation of the neuromuscular system. A magnesium deficiency hampers the proper functioning of these other nutrients.

Dosage: You need 300–350 mg of magnesium daily.

Food Sources: Magnesium is found in bran, honey, green vegetables (spinach, etc.), nuts, seafood, bone meal, and kelp tablets.

Varicose Veins

Description: These are the veins that appear on the surface of the skin. At times, they can be enlarged and twisted. Many people believe varicose veins are caused only by aging and poor circulation. However, this problem also results from a deficiency of vitamin F, whose primary function is to control blood flow. Proper blood flow leads to proper circulation, which leads to proper functioning of the blood vessels.

Dosage: There is no daily recommendation for vitamin F, but it should make up 10 percent of your total calories.

Food Sources: Vegetable oils, wheat germ, and sunflower seeds are good sources of vitamin F.

Vitiligo

Description: *Vitiligo* is a medical term that describes a condition in which the body is unable to produce melanin. The symptoms appear as light blotches on the skin. Vitiligo often occurs as a reaction to sunburn. It can also occur due to a deficiency of para-aminobenzoic acid (PABA). PABA stimulates red blood cell formation as well as restores color to cells. The result is appropriate skin color throughout the body.

Dosage: There is no specific dosage for PABA, but 10–100 mg daily is suggested .

Food Sources: PABA is supplied by blackstrap molasses, brewer's yeast, liver, organ meats, and wheat germ.

Vomiting

Description: Scientifically, vomiting is defined as the ejection of material from the stomach through the mouth. Basically, it is just upchucking food that has disagreed with you.

It is also possible that vomiting can occur from a lack of pantothenic acid and sodium. Pantothenic acid regulates the conversion of food into energy during digestion. Sodium aids in muscle contraction. Working together, these nutrients aid the digestive system by properly passing food through the gastrointestinal tract. Thus, any reverse action is prevented.

Dosage: You should have .5–10 mg of pantothenic acid a day. There is no specific requirement for sodium.

Food Sources: Pantothenic acid comes from brewer's yeast, legumes, organ meats, salmon, wheat germ, whole grains, and fresh orange juice. Sodium is found in salt, milk, cheese, and seafood.

Warts

Description: A wart is a small, usually hard, benign growth formed on and rooted in the skin. Warts tend to appear mostly on the hands, fingers, elbows, and face. The condition is caused by a virus. A lack of vitamin A makes the body more susceptible to infection. Therefore, an adequate supply of vitamin A, with its ability to help the body resist infection, will serve as a preventive if not a curative.

Dosage: You should have 5,000 IU of vitamin A daily.

Food Sources: Vitamin A is supplied by green and yellow fruits and vegetables (apricots, spinach, and raw carrots, e.g.), milk, fish liver oil, and beef liver.

Weakness

Description: Feelings of weakness involve a lack of physical strength or vigor, and they are often associated with fatigue and sluggishness. Weakness can be both a physical and a psychological phenomenon. Physically weak people are not strong. They cannot lift heavy objects or exert themselves for an extended period of time. Mentally weak people show similar characteristics. They are easily influenced by others and are unable to stick to a task.

Physical weakness, as well as mental weakness, is due to a lack of training. However, weakness is also the result of nutritional deficiencies, notably vitamins B_6 and B_{12}, niacin, copper, and potassium. These vitamins and minerals are involved in digestion, metabolism, and the production of red blood cells, which leads to nourishment of the cells. Additionally, the nutrients help regulate the neuromuscular system. This regulation can often lead to increased activity, which, in and of itself, is enough to overcome feelings of weakness.

Dosage: You need 1.8-2.2 mg of vitamin B_6, 3 mcg of B_{12}, 11-18 mg of niacin, and 2 mg of copper daily. There is no specific recommendation for potassium.

Food Sources: Vitamin B_6 is found in blackstrap molasses, brewer's yeast, green leafy vegetables, meat, organ meats, wheat germ, whole grains, dessicated liver, brown rice, and peas. Good sources of vitamin B_{12} include cheese, fish, milk, organ meats, tuna, and eggs. Niacin comes from brewer's yeast, seafood, lean meats, milk, poultry, dessicated liver, and roasted peanuts. Copper is supplied by legumes, nuts, organ meats, seafood, raisins, molasses, and bone meal. Finally, potassium occurs in dates, figs, peaches, tomato juice, blackstrap molasses, peanuts, raisins, seafood, apricots, bananas, green peppers, potatoes, and sunflower seeds.

It is obvious that many of these nutrients are found in similar foods. Therefore, a well-balanced diet that includes these foods will supply the nutrients to increase vigor.

Weight Loss

Description: The inability to maintain a constant weight, or the inexplicable dropping of weight, is usually due to a deficiency of phosphorus and sodium. These minerals aid in metabolism and muscle activity, which is secondarily related to the digestion and absorption of foodstuffs. Thus, weight will be maintained as more food is stored. Please remember that this description of weight loss refers strictly to a nutritional deficiency, not a deliberate behavioral action to lose weight.

Dosage: You should get 800 mg of phosphorus a day. While there is no standard for sodium intake, 100–300 mg per day is considered sufficient.

Food Sources: Phosphorus comes from eggs, fish, grains, glandular meats, meat, poultry, yellow cheese, milk, and yogurt. Sodium is found in salt, milk, cheese, and seafood.

Wound Healing
(Slow, Prolonged,
or Incomplete)

Description: This is not so much a symptom or a disease as it is the inability of the body to heal properly or rapidly enough. Slow healing of a wound is usually due to a lack of vitamin C and zinc. Both nutrients have as one of their many functions the proper healing of wounds. Without these nutrients in adequate supply, susceptibility to infections increases.

Dosage: You need 60 mg of vitamin C and 15 mg of zinc daily.

Food Sources: Vitamin C is supplied by citrus fruits, cantaloupe, green peppers, broccoli, and potatoes. Zinc comes from brewer's yeast, liver, seafood, soybeans, spinach, sunflower seeds, and mushrooms.

Xerophthalmia
(Lack of Tearing)

Description: The inability of the eyes to tear or to maintain an appropriate moisture level is called *xerophthalmia*. It is due to a deficiency of vitamin A that results in an absence of eye lubricants. Vitamin A regulates the hormonal and biochemical processes that produce tears and keep the eyes moist to prevent blindness.

Dosage: You need 5,000 IU of vitamin A per day.

Food Sources: Vitamin A is found in green and yellow fruits and vegetables (apricots, spinach, and raw carrots, e.g.), milk, fish liver oil, and beef liver.

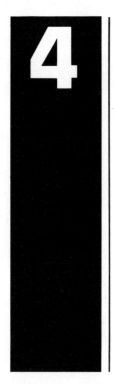

Vitamins and Minerals

The American diet is hazardous to your health. In a land where food is plentiful it is hard to believe that nutritional deficiencies can exist. But they do, and worse, they lead to deficiency symptoms. Deficiency symptoms are related to a lack of a specific vitamin or mineral. These symptoms can be a minor ache or pain or even a major illness. The question is: How and why do they occur?

We consume too much fat, too much sugar, too much caffeine, and a host of other nutritionally harmful foods. These foods do not supply the appropriate nutrients, or they prevent their absorption, or they somehow totally rob the body of vitamins and minerals. In any case, a lack of a particular nutrient, no matter how it occurs, can create an ailment or an illness. Deliberate supplementation, through pills or proper food intake, will not guarantee the prevention of a deficiency symptom, nor will it promise the cure of one. However, adequate intake of vitamins and minerals helps the body work better, and this is probably what prevents or cures a deficiency symptom. Remember, it is not the nutrient itself, but how the vitamin or mineral helps the body function more effectively, that improves the deficiency symptom.

This chapter is divided into two sections. Vitamins are listed alphabetically, with descriptions of their contribution to bodily functions, the symptoms that may arise in cases of deficiency, and the conditions that a proper intake of the vitamins may improve. The same information is given for minerals, also listed alphabetically, in the second part of this chapter.

VITAMINS

Vitamin A

Vitamin A is best known for its effects on night vision. People who have difficulty seeing in the dark are always told to consume more vitamin A because this will improve their eyesight. This is very true. In fact, the scientific term for vitamin A is *retinol,* derived from the *retina* of the eye. The retina must contain an appropriate amount of vitamin A so that the biochemical process of vision and sight can occur. Vitamin A also serves other functions. It aids the body in tissue growth and repair, thus preventing infections. Healthy skin is the first line of defense, and vitamin A promotes the growth of epithelial tissue, which covers all organs, including the skin. Second, this vitamin aids in the development of a strong immune system to protect the body against infections. A third way vitamin A serves a protective function is to act as an antioxidant. An antioxidant prevents the cell structures from combining with oxygen. Every cell needs a certain amount of oxygen to work properly, but too much oxygen will cause the cell to suffer. This has been implicated in the aging process, so it is possible that vitamin A may serve another function, that of retarding aging.

Vitamin A has also recently been shown to be effective in the treatment of cancer. This does not mean that enough or extra doses of vitamin A will prevent cancer, nor does it mean that a deficiency of vitamin A will cause cancer. It simply means that some evidence has accumulated to indicate that this vitamin has a beneficial effect in the treatment of cancer, probably by boosting the power of the immune system. (Remember, vitamin A is a fat-soluble vitamin that is stored in the body. Therefore, excessive intake can create toxicity. However, a lack of vitamin A will cause a number of deficiency symptoms.)

A deficiency of vitamin A can cause many problems. Some of these symptoms include allergies, loss of appetite, acne, blemishes, dry hair, arthritis, asthma, fatigue, itching or burning eyes, athlete's foot, bronchitis, colds, cystitis, loss of smell, diabetes, eczema, night blindness, rough skin, hepatitis, migraines, sinus troubles, psoriasis, soft teeth, and susceptibility to infection. This list, though wide-ranging is incomplete. Cancer was omitted deliberately because the relationship between vitamin A and cancer is still tenuous. However, studies have shown that people with adequate to high intakes of vitamin A have a lower likelihood of getting cancer than people who are deficient. Other symptoms may also have been omitted, but the most common ones are listed above.

The easiest way to ensure that you are getting enough vitamin A is to take a supplement. This is true with any vitamin or mineral. The main drawback is that it becomes expensive. The other way, and probably the best way to get all your vitamins and minerals, is from the foods you eat. Vitamin A is primarily supplied by green and yellow fruits and vegetables (apricots, spinach, and raw carrots, e.g.), milk, fish liver oil, and beef liver. If these items are not part of your daily diet, then perhaps a change in food choices is necessary.

Vitamin A is one of several vitamins which, when taken in

excessive doses, can have a toxic or poisonous effect on the body. Because vitamin A is fat soluble, it is stored in the body, and builds up over a period of time. However, as long as you stay within a safe range (see appendix), you needn't worry about the toxicity of vitamin A.

A vitamin A overdose usually manifests itself in skin color, which takes on a yellow-orange tint. Prolonged, excessive intake can also lead to hair loss, nausea, headaches, skin problems, fatigue, appetite loss, muscle weakness, bone and joint pain, and an enlargement of the liver and spleen. Ironically, many of these toxicity symptoms closely resemble the deficiency symptoms of the same vitamin. Clearly, too much or too little of vitamin A is not healthy.

B COMPLEX VITAMINS

The B complex vitamins are a collection of nutrients grouped together because they serve similar functions. These vitamins are mainly responsible for metabolism and energy production. They fulfill this responsibility by contributing to the function of the circulatory, digestive, muscular, and nervous systems. A list of the B vitamins include B_1 (thiamine), B_2 (riboflavin), B_6 (pyridoxine), B_{12} (cobalamin), biotin, choline, folic acid, inositol, niacin, pangamic acid (B_{15}), pantothenic acid, and para-aminobenzoic acid (PABA). Laetrile, also known as B_{17}, is not discussed here because the Food and Drug Administration has banned its use in the United States.

The B complex vitamins are very important to good health. These vitamins are water-soluble, which means they cannot be stored in the body. They are excreted through perspiration and urine, and therefore, they must be replaced daily. The B complex vitamins, along with vitamin C, are also considered antistress vitamins because of their positive effects on the nervous system.

Vitamin B₁ (Thiamine)

Thiamine is a vitamin that affects almost every major organ in the body: the brain, heart, ears, eyes, stomach and nervous system. It is also a coenzyme that regulates the metabolism and aids in the absorption of neurotransmitters. This latter function allows the nervous system and the brain to operate properly. Vitamin B_1 also aids the body's digestive processes, circulation, and energy production. Deficiencies of vitamin B_1 are now rare, but if they do occur, major problems can result.

The most well-known thiamine deficiency is beriberi, a disease of the peripheral nervous system. Other deficiency symptoms include appetite loss, alcoholism, anemia, congestive heart failure, constipation, digestive disturbances, diarrhea, fatigue, irritability, nervousness, nausea, numbness of hands and feet, shortness of breath, rapid heart rate, and increased susceptibility to stress.

These symptoms can be prevented simply by assuring adequate intake of vitamin B_1 through food sources. These include blackstrap molasses, brewer's yeast, brown rice, fish, meat, nuts, organ meats, poultry, wheat germ, and sunflower seeds. Remember, this vitamin, and all the other B complex vitamins, cannot be stored. Therefore, you must provide for their intake every day.

Vitamin B₂ (Riboflavin)

Riboflavin is the soft body tissue vitamin. It mainly affects the eyes, hair, nails, and skin by improving metabolism, red blood cell formation, and cell respiration. Cells must breathe to function properly, and vitamin B_2 is absolutely vital for this to occur.

When there are insufficient amounts of riboflavin, specific deficiency symptoms occur. These include cataracts, cracks in the corners of the mouth, sores in the mouth, dizziness, itching and burning eyes, digestive problems, retarded growth, a red sore tongue, acne, alcoholism, arthritis, athlete's foot, baldness, diarrhea, and excessive reaction to stress. Adequate amounts of vitamin B_2 will help improve these conditions, but there is no guarantee that the vitamin will totally cure the symptoms.

The best way to prevent B_2 deficiencies from occurring is to eat foods rich in this vitamin. These include blackstrap molasses, nuts, organ meats, whole grains, almonds, Brussels sprouts, and brewer's yeast.

Vitamin B_6 (Pyridoxine)

Pyridoxine is one of the most versatile of the B complex vitamins. It improves the function of the blood, muscles, nerves, and skin. It also aids in antibody formation, digestion, and weight control. More specifically, vitamin B_6 is a preventative in heart disease, menstrual problems, complications of pregnancy, and birth defects. The vitamin also acts as a coenzyme in the breakdown and conversion of amino acids. For example, tryptophan cannot be converted to niacin unless vitamin B_6 is present.

The vitamin is so beneficial to human health that a lack of it causes wide-ranging deficiency symptoms. Some of these include acne, anemia, arthritis, atherosclerosis, baldness, high serum cholesterol, convulsions in babies, cystitis, depression, dizziness, hair loss, hypoglycemia, irritability, learning disabilities, mental retardation, muscular disorders, nervous disorders, nausea, weight problems, weakness, and sensitivity to stress. Remember, the vitamin is not a cure-all for these symptoms, but it may prevent their occurrence or lessen their effect.

Vitamin B_6 is found in many of the same foods as the other B complex vitamins. These are blackstrap molasses, brewer's yeast, green leafy vegetables, meat, organ meats, wheat germ, whole grains, dessicated liver, prunes, brown rice, and peas.

Vitamin B_{12} (Cobalamin)

Cobalamin is the only vitamin to contain a metal, cobalt. It is a very large and complex molecule because of this. Vitamin B_{12} serves several essential functions, including blood cell formation, maintenance of appetite through its regulatory effect on metabolism, maintenance of a healthy nervous system, and an increase in cellular life. Cobalamin can be absorbed by the body only in the presence of a glycoprotein substance called the *intrinsic factor*. A deficiency of B_{12} is usually caused by a lack of the intrinsic factor, thus preventing absorption, rather than by a dietary lack of the vitamin.

Deficiency symptoms are evidenced as alcoholism, allergies, anemia, arthritis, bronchial asthma, bursitis, fatigue, hypoglycemia, insomnia, nervousness, shingles, stress reactions, walking and speaking difficulties, and weight problems. Other deficiency symptoms include the impaired function of the small intestine (absorption problems), a delay in blood clotting, and visual difficulties along with reduced color perception.

The best food sources of vitamin B_{12} are cheese, fish, milk, organ meats, tuna, eggs, and cottage cheese.

Biotin

Biotin is a unique vitamin within the B complex family. One of its functions is to promote the utilization of the other B complex vitamins. Additionally, biotin regulates cell growth, fatty acid production, and metabolism. Furthermore, the thyroid gland and the adrenal glands depend on this vitamin to maintain proper function. Thus, biotin is a major factor in the body's production and use of energy.

Biotin deficiencies are manifested in very specific symptoms. Severe dermatitis and hair loss leading to baldness are the most common. Other symptoms include depression, dry skin, eczema, fatigue, grayish skin color, insomnia, leg cramps, muscular pain and weakness, and a poor appetite.

Adequate intake of biotin-rich foods can resolve a deficiency. Some of them are legumes, whole grains, organ meats, brewer's yeast, lentils, egg yolk, and soybeans.

Choline

Choline is considered part of the B complex vitamins because it occurs in conjunction with so many of these vitamins. Although choline's role as a coenzyme is sometimes questioned, the vitamin does have positive effects on the hair, kidneys, liver, and thymus gland. Choline also promotes lecithin formation, metabolism, and nerve transmission, and regulates the liver and gall bladder.

Many deficiency symptoms are associated with a lack of choline. These include alcoholism, atherosclerosis, baldness, bleeding stomach ulcers, high serum cholesterol, constipation, dizziness, ear noises, headaches, high blood pressure, hypoglycemia, impaired liver and kidney function, and insomnia. These conditions can be improved by adequate intake of choline.

Some of the best food sources of choline are brewer's yeast, fish, legumes, organ meats, soybeans, wheat germ, lecithin, egg yolks, and peanuts.

Folic Acid (Folacin)

Folic acid primarily affects the blood, glands, and liver. The vitamin is also necessary for the synthesis of DNA and RNA. Thus, those organs that depend on the rapid reproduction of new cells, such as bone marrow, fingernails, hair, the immune system, and red blood cells, are aided by folic acid. Folic acid also maintains appetite and metabolism and is primary in the production of red blood cells.

A folacin deficiency can lead to alcholism, anemia, atherosclerosis, baldness, diarrhea, digestive problems, fatigue, graying hair, growth problems, menstrual problems, mental illness, stomach ulcers, and stress. Other deficiency symptoms include weakness; an inflamed, sore tongue; numbness or tingling in the hands and feet; depression; irritability; pallor; drowsiness; and a slow, weakened pulse. Usually these latter symptoms occur only in severe deficiency cases.

Folic acid is provided in the diet by many common foods. Some of them are green leafy vegetables (spinach, etc.), milk, organ meats, oysters, salmon, whole grains, brewer's yeast, dates, and tuna fish. Remember, ingestion of folic acid does not guarantee the cure of any of these conditions, but it can possibly improve them and prevent some of them.

Inositol

Inositol is another of the versatile B complex vitamins that affects several major organs. The brain, hair, heart, kidneys, liver, and muscles all benefit from adequate amounts of inositol. (Although there is no specific recommended daily dosage, the suggested range for inositol intake is 100–1,000 mg.) Inositol seems to function chiefly as a protective mechanism against heart disease. Inositol retards hardening of the arteries, reduces cholesterol, aids in the formation of lecithin, and promotes the metabolism of fats and cholesterol.

It is obvious that some of the deficiency symptoms related to inositol would concern the heart. These include high serum cholesterol, atherosclerosis, and the promotion of heart disease. Other deficiency symptoms are constipation, baldness, eczema, eye problems, hair loss, and obesity.

Inositol is found in many foods. The major sources are blackstrap molasses, citrus fruits, brewer's yeast, meat, milk, nuts, vegetables, whole grains, and lecithin.

Niacin (B$_3$)

Niacin is one of the most well known, yet most controversial, of all the B complex vitamins. It has been used to treat everything from heart disease to arthritis to mental illness to alcoholism. This is because niacin is necessary for the proper function of the brain, liver, nerves, and skin. While niacin does have a positive effect on these organs and the above conditions, it is by no means a cure-all. In fact, the major sign of a niacin deficiency is not related to any of those conditions.

Pellagra is the primary niacin deficiency symptom. Pellagra

is characterized by the three Ds: dermatitis, diarrhea, and dementia. Other signs of niacin deficiency include acne, appetite loss, canker sores, depression, halitosis, fatigue, headaches, high blood pressure, indigestion, insomnia, leg cramps, poor circulation, muscular weakness, nausea, stress reactions, nervous disorders, skin eruptions, and tooth decay. Often, a deficiency cannot be compensated for with the recommended doses of niacin. Rather, megadoses may be needed, but you should check with your physician first.

Niacin deficiencies can be prevented by eating foods rich in this vitamin. Some of them are brewer's yeast, seafood, lean meats, milk, poultry, dessicated liver, rhubarb, and peanuts. You can also get niacin from dried peas, beans, nuts, and whole grains.

Pangamic Acid (B_{15})

Pangamic acid was once thought to be the answer to an endurance athlete's problems. Ingestion of B_{15} would increase endurance and sustain performance over long periods of time. While this may be true, it is likely to be a secondary result of pangamic acid's primary functions. This vitamin helps regulate the activity of the glands, heart, kidneys, and nerves, while improving metabolic processes and cell oxidation and respiration. A lack of B_{15} can lead to some major deficiency symptoms.

A pangamic acid deficiency may be evidenced by alcoholism, asthma, atherosclerosis, high cholesterol, emphysema, heart disease, headaches, insomnia, poor circulation, premature aging, nervous and glandular disorders, rheumatism, and shortness of breath.

Pangamic acid is found in brewer's yeast; brown rice; rare meat; sunflower, pumpkin, and sesame seeds; whole grains; and organ meats. Once again, you must remember that supplying your body with vitamin B_{15} does not mean you can cure a deficiency symptom. You may improve on it only to the point at which you are healthy enough to function effectively.

Pantothenic Acid (Pantothenate)

Pantothenic acid is the essential part of coenzyme A, which is responsible for cellular metabolism. Thus, every cell in the body depends on pantothenic acid. Additionally, the adrenal glands are very dependent on this vitamin for proper functioning. Therefore, the body's entire response to stress can be affected by the amount of pantothenate in the system. Finally, pantothenic acid improves the functions of the digestive system, the nervous system, and the skin.

Deficiencies of this vitamin lead to a variety of symptoms. Some of them are allergies, arthritis, baldness, cystitis, diarrhea, digestive disorders, duodenal ulcers, eczema, hypoglycemia, intestinal disorders, kidney trouble, loss of hair, muscle cramps, premature aging, respiratory infections, restlessness, sore feet, stress reactions, tooth decay, and vomiting.

The best food sources of pantothenic acid include brewer's yeast, legumes, organ meats, salmon, wheat germ, whole grains, mushrooms, and orange juice.

Para-aminobenzoic Acid (PABA)

PABA is probably best known for its use as a sunscreen in suntan lotions, but it serves other vital functions as well. It promotes glandular activity, hair color restoration, intestinal activity, and blood cell formation. PABA is also essential for keeping the skin healthy.

Deficiency disorders related to PABA are not very common, but they can occur. They include constipation, baldness, depression, digestive disorders, fatigue, gray hair, headaches, irritability, overactive thyroid, rheumatic fever, stress reactivity, sunburn, wrinkles, and, in some cases, infertility.

These conditions can be improved by ingesting 10–100 mg of PABA daily. This is a suggested range since there is no recommended daily dosage. The best food sources of PABA are blackstrap molasses, brewer's yeast, liver, organ meats, and wheat germ.

Vitamin C (Ascorbic Acid)

Vitamin C is probably the most well known of all the vitamins. People have taken it to cure everything from the common cold to cancer. While vitamin C does play some very important roles in human health, it is not a wonder drug or a miracle cure. Vitamin C has some very specific effects on the body.

First, vitamin C has a beneficial effect on the functioning of many organs, such as the adrenal glands, blood system, connective tissue, gums, teeth, and heart. Second, vitamin C plays a vital role in cellular respiration and the metabolism of amino acids. Third, this vitamin is necessary for the formation of collagen and other fibrous connective tissue. Fourth, and probably the most well known, is the ability of vitamin C to strengthen the immune system and increase the body's resistance to infections, especially colds. The major drawback of vitamin C is that it is water-soluble and cannot be stored by the body. Therefore you must supply your body with it every day.

If you do not receive enough vitamin C, deficiency symptoms and even major illnesses can occur. Volumes have been written on vitamin C and its relation to cancer, diabetes, heart disease, arthritis, and many other major diseases. Adequate intake, and even megadoses, will not guarantee a cure from or even prevention of these diseases. The same holds true for the other, and sometimes less serious, deficiency symptoms associated with vitamin C. These include scurvy, alchoholism, allergies, anemia, atherosclerosis, baldness, bleeding gums, capillary wall rupture, high serum cholesterol, colds, susceptibility to bruises, dental cavities, cystitis, hypoglycemia, hepatitis, overweight, nosebleeds, prickly heat, sinusitis, tooth decay, poor digestion, and increased susceptibility to stress. This list is extensive but not totally inclusive. If one of these symptoms does occur, excessive vitamin C is not always the answer. Because some is good, more is not always better.

It is best to get your supply of vitamin C from its food sources. These are citrus fruits, cantaloupe, green peppers, broccoli, and potatoes. Other sources include cauliflower, tomatoes, Brussels sprouts, and bean sprouts. Never underestimate the importance of this vitamin to your health, but don't overestimate its capabilities, either.

Vitamin D

Vitamin D has been called the "sunshine vitamin" because the body can synthesize it in the presence of sunlight. People have also mistakenly classified vitamin D as necessary only for children to build strong bones and teeth. The truth is that vitamin D is equally important for adults.

Vitamin D helps build strong cartilage, bones, and teeth by allowing the body to absorb calcium and phosphorus. The vitamin also regulates heart action, maintains nervous system functioning, improves skin respiration, and regulates the thyroid gland. With these roles to play, it is easy to see why vitamin D is important to people of all ages.

A lack of vitamin D results in some very specific deficiency symptoms. These include a burning sensation in the mouth and throat; acne; alcoholism; allergies; arthritis; cystitis; diarrhea; eczema; insomnia; myopia; nervousness; poor metabolism; psoriasis; soft bones, teeth, and connective tissue; and stress reactivity. Some other, and perhaps better known, vitamin D deficiencies are rickets, osteomalacia, osteoporosis, and possibly kidney disease.

However, you *can* have too much of a good thing. Excessive doses of vitamin D can increase blood levels of calcium and phosphorus, and redeposit them in the soft tissues of the blood vessels, kidneys, heart and lungs. This can lead to the calcification and possible deterioration of these organs. Other symptoms of toxicity include appetite loss, diarrhea, headaches, thirst, urgency to urinate, and vomiting.

Since vitamin D can be synthesized by the body in the presence of sunlight, deficiency symptoms are somewhat rare. They do occur, however, so it is best to tilt the odds in your favor by eating foods rich in vitamin D. Some of these are egg yolks, organ meats, bone meal, milk, yogurt, salmon, tuna fish, and other foods fortified with vitamin D.

Vitamin E

Vitamin E has probably had more nicknames than any other vitamin. It has been called the "sex vitamin," the "heart vitamin," and the "antiaging vitamin." Vitamin E is related to the function of these systems and processes, but the nicknames are more the result of good publicity than the result of miracle powers.

Vitamin E works as an antioxidant, so it may very well slow the aging process since cell oxidation speeds up as we grow older. The vitamin also works on the blood vessels and the heart by increasing blood flow to the heart, strengthening the capillary walls, and reducing serum cholesterol. Vitamin E works within the reproductive system to increase fertility and male potency and within the respiratory system to protect the lungs from pollutants. This vitamin also has positive effects on pituitary gland function, the skin, and the muscles and nerves.

With all these benefits, it is hard to believe that any vitamin E deficiency could exist. Unfortunately, deficiencies can occur. One of vitamin E's main functions is to protect cells, especially polyunsaturated fatty acids (PFA), from oxidation. However, the more PFA in the diet, the more vitamin E is needed. It is almost a "catch 22," since you need to eat PFAs to protect against heart disease. Thus, if you do not properly alter your food intake to supply sufficient amounts of vitamin E, deficiency symptoms can occur. These include allergies, arthritis, atherosclerosis, baldness, high serum cholesterol, cystitis, dry (dull or falling) hair, diabetes, enlarged prostate, heart disease, impotence, menstrual problems, miscarriages, migraines, muscular wasting, myopia, overweight, phlebitis, sinusitis, stress, sterility, thrombosis, varicose veins, warts, and wrinkles.

Vitamin E is fat-soluble and can be stored in the body. However, there have been very few reports of toxicity, probably due to all the vitamin's functions. You should note that certain people should not take vitamin E without a doctor's approval: people with high blood pressure, insulin-dependent diabetes, and hypothyroidism. Supplementation is possible, but it is recommended that you receive vitamin E from its food sources. These are dark green vegetables, eggs, liver, organ meats, wheat germ, vegetable oils, oatmeal, peanuts, and tomatoes.

Vitamin F

Vitamin F is sort of a pseudovitamin. Vitamin F stands for the unsaturated fatty acids that we must eat to preserve cellular function. Vitamin F also improves the functions of the glands, hair, mucous membranes, nerves, and skin. This vitamin is essential to the prevention of hardening of the arteries and to improving blood coagulation, normalizing blood pressure, destroying serum cholesterol, and stimulating growth and vital organ respiration.

The deficiency symptoms associated with vitamin F include acne, allergies, baldness, bronchial asthma, high serum cholesterol, diarrhea, dry skin, dry hair, eczema, gall bladder problems, heart disease, leg ulcers, nail problems, psoriasis, weight problems, and varicose veins. These symptoms can be improved or possibly prevented by eating foods rich in vitamin D such as vegetable oils, wheat germ, and sunflower seeds.

Vitamin K (Menadione)

Vitamin K gets its name from the Scandinavian word *koagulation*, which describes its function. The vitamin promotes blood clotting by working through the blood system and the liver to form the precursors of thrombin, which is the active agent in the clotting of the blood.

Deficiencies of vitamin K are rare in adults because the vitamin can be synthesized by intestinal bacteria. Unfortunately, deficiencies can occur in newborns because they have no intestinal bacteria. If a deficiency is present, the symptoms to look for include diarrhea, increased tendency to hemorrhage, bruising, gallstones, menstrual problems, miscarriages, and nosebleeds. As you can see, the major problem related to vitamin K deficiency is bleeding.

In addition to being synthesized, vitamin K is supplied by green leafy vegetables, safflower oil, blackstrap molasses, yogurt, oatmeal, and beef liver.

MINERALS

Calcium

Calcium is the most important mineral in the body. The hardness and strength of the bones, teeth, and cartilage depend on calcium. While calcium is stored in these structures, it is also exchanged daily in the body fluids. If your dietary intake is below desired levels, the fluids extract calcium from the bones and it is not replaced.

Calcium is so important to so many organs in the body that there is talk of raising the recommended daily allowance from 800 mg to 1,400 mg. In addition to the bones, teeth, and soft connective tissue, the heart, skin, blood, and nervous system depend on calcium to function properly. This mineral aids in blood clotting, controlling heart rhythm, stimulating muscle growth and contraction, and tranquilizing and maintaining the transmissions of the nervous system.

Calcium deficiencies are not as rare as you might think. They can occur due to a lack of calcium or an inability to absorb the mineral into the system. In either case deficiency symptoms can lead to both major and minor problems. These include arthritis, aging signs (backache, bone pain, finger tremors), foot and leg cramps, heart palpitations, insomnia, menstrual cramps, muscle cramps, nervousness, limb numbness, premenstrual tension, rheumatism, tooth decay, and weight problems. The other major deficiency symptom associated with calcium is osteoporosis.

These symptoms can be improved or possibly prevented through adequate intake of calcium. To give you an idea of how much calcium is necessary, you need to drink a quart of milk a day, every day, just to get the minimum required dosage. Other food sources include cheese, molasses, yogurt, bone meal, dolomite, almonds, and beef liver. If you cannot eat these foods, the supplementation is necessary.

Chromium

The amount of chromium needed by the body is very small. However, the job this mineral performs is very large. Chromium serves as a coenzyme to insulin in the metabolism of sugars. Other metabolic processes are also improved in the presence of chromium. Additionally, chromium may help reduce cholesterol levels and the incidence of plaque.

A deficiency of chromium can lead to major illnesses. These are diabetes, hypoglycemia, and atherosclerosis. It is essential that your diet provide enough chromium. Although there is no recommended daily dosage, and the suggested range is 100–300 mcg, the National Research Council says that up to 2 mg a day will be safe and effective. You can achieve these chromium intake levels by eating brewer's yeast, clams, corn oil, and whole grain cereals.

Copper

Copper is an important component in the function of several systems of the body, including the formation of hemoglobin and red blood cells, the healing processes of the body, and bone formation. It also will improve skin tone as well as the texture and growth of hair. Also, the myelin sheaths that cover nerve fibers depend on copper to function effectively.

Only a few deficiency symptoms are associated with a lack of this mineral: anemia, baldness, general weakness, impaired respiration, and skin sores. Most, if not all of them, can be improved through adequate intake. The best food sources of copper are legumes, nuts, organ meats, seafood, raisins, molasses, bone meal, and soybeans.

Iodine

Iodine has long been considered the mineral necessary for proper thyroid function. This is true, but iodine also facilitates the actions of body metabolism, energy production, and general physical and mental development, including the growth of hair, nails, healthy skin, and teeth.

A deficiency of iodine causes the thyroid gland to work harder, thus becoming enlarged. This condition is known as *goiter*. Other symptoms caused by a lack of iodine are cold hands and feet, dry hair, atherosclerosis, irritability, nervousness, and obesity. Interestingly, an excess of iodine creates the same physiological effects as a deficiency. This hyperthyroidism leads to a speeded-up metabolism and may even cause acne.

The best food sources of iodine are seafood, kelp tablets, and iodized salt; but remember to watch your consumption of salt.

Iron

Iron prevents "tired blood," as the television commercials used to say. Iron is the primary component in the hemoglobin of red blood cells, and it is responsible for transporting oxygen to all the body's cells. Iron also helps the body resist stress and disease and improves the structure of the bones, nails, skin, and teeth.

The most common deficiency symptom associated with iron is anemia. Other symptoms include alcoholism, breathing difficulties, brittle nails, colitis, constipation, and menstrual problems. It is fairly easy to remedy these conditions by consuming iron-rich foods, such as blackstrap molasses, eggs, fish, organ meats, poultry, wheat germ, dessicated liver, dried beans and fruits, and green leafy vegetables.

Magnesium

Magnesium is more important to the body than we realize. This mineral helps regulate all cellular metabolic processes. And in proper balance with calcium, magnesium controls the functions of cardiac and skeletal muscles and nerve transmissions. The combined effect of these two minerals makes it easy to see why magnesium is also important to the structure and function of bones, teeth, heart, muscles, and nerves.

Magnesium deficiency symptoms tend to be both psychological and physical. Some of these symptoms are confusion, disorientation, anger, depression, nervousness, alcoholism, high serum cholesterol, kidney stones, prostate trouble, rapid pulse, noise sensitivity, stomach acidity, overweight, tooth decay, and tremors.

These symptoms may be counteracted by eating foods rich in magnesium, such as bran, honey, green vegetables (spinach, etc.), nuts, seafood, bone meal, kelp tablets, and tuna fish.

Manganese

Manganese serves many functions. It improves the efficiency of the brain, mammary glands, muscles, and nerves. Manganese also aids sex hormone production, tissue repair and growth, metabolism, utilization of vitamin E, and the synthesis of proteins, DNA, and RNA.

Some of the deficiency symptoms related to manganese are ataxia (muscle coordination failure), dizziness, allergies, asthma, diabetes, fatigue, and hearing difficulties. The symptoms are usually resolved by eating foods containing manganese. These include bananas, bran, celery, cereals, egg yolks, green leafy vegetables, legumes, liver, nuts, pineapples, and whole grains.

Phosphorus

Phosphorus serves more functions in the body than any other mineral. It combines with calcium to provide strong bones and teeth. It regulates cell growth and repair, metabolic and energy production processes, heart muscle contraction (with calcium), kidney function, nerve and muscle activity (also with calcium), vitamin utilization, and brain functions.

Phosphorus is so plentiful in the environment that we should be concerned more with toxicity than with deficiencies. However, while toxic levels of phosphorus are still unknown, deficiency symptoms are known. These include appetite loss, arthritis, fatigue, irregular breathing, nervous disorders, stunted growth in children, stress, tooth and gum disorders, and weight problems.

The best food sources of phosphorus are eggs, fish, grains, glandular meats, meat, poultry, yellow cheese, calf liver, milk, and yogurt.

Potassium

Potassium is very abundant in the human body. It regulates heartbeat, muscle contraction, nervous system excitability, blood flow, and kidney function. Potassium also serves as a counterbalance to sodium in keeping blood pressure low.

Potassium deficiencies can occur despite the availability of this mineral. People on low-calorie diets are very susceptible to potassium deficiencies. Some of the symptoms include acne; alcoholism; allergies; colic in infants; continuous thirst; diabetes; dry skin; constipation; general weakness; high blood pressure; insomnia; muscle damage; heart disease; nervousness; slow, irregular heartbeat; and slow reflexes.

There are many common, everyday foods that supply potassium, so you should be able to prevent a deficiency from occurring. Potassium-rich foods are dates, figs, peaches, tomato juice, blackstrap molasses, peanuts, raisins, seafood, apricots, bananas, green peppers, potatoes, sunflower seeds, broccoli, squash, fresh fruits, and orange juice.

Selenium

Selenium is a mineral that only recently has received its due. Selenium acts as a preventer of heart disease and cancer and also aids vitamin E as an antioxidant. This mineral is also involved in cellular respiration, energy transfer, sperm cell production, pancreatic function, and antibody synthesis. Selenium contributes to the maintenance of muscle cells and red blood cells.

Deficiency symptoms associated with a lack of selenium include heart disease and cancer; however, it is important to note that a selenium deficiency does not necessarily cause these diseases.

The food sources of selenium include brewer's yeast, organ meats, seafood, and whole grains. Foods high in fat or sugar are usually low in selenium.

Sodium

Sodium is a very plentiful mineral that serves a very important function. Its main purpose is to regulate fluid levels in cells and to aid in muscle contraction through a mechanism called the *sodium pump*. This mineral also plays a role in maintaining the integrity of the lymphatic and nervous systems.

Everyone is aware that too much sodium can lead to an increase in blood pressure and water retention. Unfortunately, people are unaware that sodium deficiencies can lead to conditions that may also be harmful. Some of these deficiency symptoms are appetite loss, dehydration, fever, heat stroke, intestinal gas, muscle shrinkage, vomiting, and weight loss. It is ironic that either extreme of this mineral can cause problems, considering the important role sodium plays in body functions.

Sodium is supplied in salt, cheese, milk, and seafood, and it is hidden in many canned and processed foods as a preservative.

Zinc

Zinc is so versatile and necessary a mineral that some people want to classify it as a vitamin. Zinc has been identified as a cofactor in more than 40 different enzyme systems and reactions. Zinc is involved in the synthesis of DNA and RNA and in the metabolism of protein. The mineral is also necessary for cell growth and the formation of connective tissue. Other processes that are facilitated by zinc are burns and wound healing; carbohydrate metabolism; prostate gland function; reproductive organ growth, development, and maturity; and vitamin B_1 and phosphorus metabolism.

With all these functions, it is easy to see why zinc is so important. A lack of the mineral can lead to a host of deficiency symptoms, including alcoholism; atherosclerosis; baldness; cirrhosis; delayed sexual maturity; diabetes; fatigue; loss of taste; poor appetite; prolonged wound healing; retarded growth; sterility; high serum cholesterol; skin lesions; birth deformities (in children if mothers are deficient); impaired development of muscular, nervous, and skeletal systems; decreased absorption of other nutrients; increased stress reactivity; and weakened immune system response.

The best way to attempt to prevent or improve any of these deficiencies is to eat foods that supply zinc, including brewer's yeast, liver, seafood, soybeans, spinach, sunflower seeds, milk, mushrooms, legumes, nuts, and eggs.

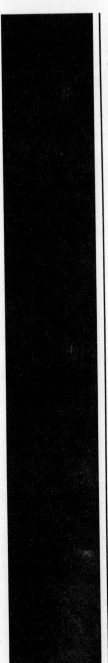

Appendix:
Vitamin and
Mineral Charts

Vitamin	Daily Dosage	Sources	Deficiency Symptoms
A Fat Soluble	RDA 5,000 IU SR 10,000–25,000 IU Toxicity 50,000 IU	Green & yellow fruits & vegetables, milk, milk products, fish liver oil, apricots (dried), liver (beef), spinach (cooked), carrots (raw)	Acne, allergies, appetite loss, arthritis, asthma, athlete's foot, blemishes, bronchitis, colds, cystitis, dry hair, eczema, fatigue, heart disease, hepatitis, itching/burning eyes, loss of smell, migraine headaches, night blindness, psoriasis, rough dry skin, sinusitis, stress, susceptibility to infections, tooth & gum disorders
B Complex	RDA see B vitamins SR see B vitamins Toxicity not known	Brewer's yeast, liver, whole grains	Acne, anemia, allergies, baldness, constipation, cystitis, digestive disturbances, fatigue, hair (dull, dry, falling), heart abnormalities, hypoglycemia, insomnia, Meniere's syndrome, menstrual difficulties, migraine headaches, overweight, postoperative nausea, skin (dry, rough), stress
B1 Thiamine Water Soluble	RDA 1–1.5 mg SR 2–10 mg Toxicity not known	Blackstrap molasses, brewer's yeast, brown rice, fish, meat, nuts, organ meats, poultry, wheat germ, peanuts, sunflower seeds, Brazil nuts	Appetite loss, congestive heart failure, constipation, diabetes, diarrhea, digestive disturbances, fatigue, irritability, indigestion, mental illness, nausea, nervousness, numbness of hands & feet, rapid heart rate, pain & noise sensitivity, pains around heart, shortness of breath, stress
B2 Riboflavin Water Soluble	RDA 1.3–1.7 mg SR 2–10 mg Toxicity not known	Blackstrap molasses, nuts, organ meats, whole grains, almonds, brussel sprouts, brewer's yeast, beef liver	Acne, arthritis, athlete's foot, baldness, cataracts, corner of mouth cracks & sores, diabetes, diarrhea, dizziness, indigestion, itching/burning eyes, retarded growth, red sore tongue

KEY: RDA — Recommended Daily Allowance   Mg — Milligrams
IU — International Units   Mcg — Micrograms
SR — Supplementary Ranges

Vitamin	Daily Dosage	Sources	Deficiency Symptoms
B6 Pyridoxine Water Soluble	RDA 1.8–2.2 mg SR 4–50 mg Toxicity not known	Blackstrap molasses, brewer's yeast, green leafy vegetables, meat, organ meats, wheat germ, whole grains, dessicated liver, liver (beef), prunes (cooked), brown rice, peas	Acne, anemia, arthritis, atherosclerosis, baldness, convulsions in babies, cystitis, depression, dizziness, facial oiliness, hair loss, hypoglycemia, irritability, learning disabilities, mental retardation, muscular disorders, nervous disorders, nausea in pregnancy, obesity, post-operative nausea, sun sensitivity, weakness
B12 Cobalamin Water Soluble	RDA 3 mcg SR 5–50 mcg Toxicity not known	Cheese, fish, milk, milk products, organ meats, cottage cheese, liver, tuna fish (canned), eggs	Allergies, anemia, arthritis, bronchial asthma, bursitis, epilepsy, fatigue, general weakness, hypoglycemia, insomnia, nervousness, pernicious anemia, obesity, shingles, walking & speaking difficulties
Biotin B Complex Water Soluble	RDA 150–300 mcg SR 300–500 mcg Toxicity not known	Legumes, whole grains, organ meats, brewer's yeast, lentils, mungbean sprouts, egg yolk, beef liver, soybeans	Baldness, depression, dermatitis, dry skin, eczema, fatigue, grayish skin color, insomnia, leg cramps, muscular pain, poor appetite
Choline B Complex Water Soluble	RDA none stated SR 100–1,000 mg Toxicity not known	Brewer's yeast, fish, legumes, organ meats, soybeans, wheat germ, lecithin, liver (beef), egg yolks, peanuts (roasted with skin)	Atherosclerosis, baldness, bleeding stomach ulcers, constipation, dizziness, ear noises, growth problems, hardening of the arteries, headaches, heart trouble, high blood pressure, hypoglycemia, impaired liver & kidney function, insomnia, intolerance to fats

Vitamin	Daily Dosage	Sources	Deficiency Symptoms
Folic Acid Folacin Water Soluble	RDA 400 mcg SR 1,000–10,000 mcg Toxicity not known	Green leafy vegetables, milk, milk products, organ meats, oysters, salmon, whole grains, brewer's yeast, dates (dried), spinach (steamed), tuna fish (canned)	Anemia, atherosclerosis, baldness, diarrhea, digestive disturbances, fatigue, graying hair, growth problems, menstrual problems, mental illness, stomach ulcers
Inositol B Complex Water Soluble	RDA none stated SR 100–1,000 mg Toxicity not known	Blackstrap molasses, citrus fruits, brewer's yeast, meat, milk, nuts, vegetables, whole grains, lecithin, peanuts (roasted with skin)	Atherosclerosis, baldness, constipation, eczema, eye abnormalities, hair loss, heart disease, obesity
Niacin Niacina-mide B Complex Water Soluble	RDA 13–18 mg SR 50–5,000 mg Toxicity not known	Brewer's yeast, seafood, lean meats, milk, milk products, poultry, dessicated liver, rhubarb (cooked), chicken (breast, fried), peanuts (roasted with skin)	Acne, appetite loss, baldness, canker sores, depression, diarrhea, fatigue, halitosis, headaches, high blood pressure, indigestion, insomnia, leg cramps, migraine headaches, muscular weakness, nausea, nervous disorders, poor circulation, skin eruptions, stress, tooth decay
Pantothenic Acid B Complex Water Soluble	RDA 0.5–10 mg SR 20–100 mg Toxicity not known	Brewer's yeast, legumes, organ meats, salmon, wheat germ, whole grains, liver (beef), mushrooms (cooked), elderberries (raw), orange juice (fresh)	Allergies, arthritis, baldness, cystitis, diarrhea, duodenal ulcers, digestive disorders, eczema, hypoglycema, intestinal disorders, kidney troubles, loss of hair, muscle cramps, premature aging, respiratory infections, restlessness, nerve problems, sore feet, vomiting, tooth decay

Vitamin	Daily Dosage		Sources	Deficiency Symptoms
Para Amino-benzoic Acid Paba B Complex Water Soluble	RDA SR Toxicity	none stated 10–100 mg —	Blackstrap molasses, brewer's yeast, liver, organ meats, wheat germ	Baldness, constipation, depression, digestive disorders, dry skin, fatigue, graying hair, headaches, infertility, overactive thyroid, rheumatic fever, dark skin spots, sunburn
Pangamic B15 Water Soluble	RDA SR Toxicity	none stated not known not known	Brewer's yeast, brown rice, meat (rare), seeds (sunflower, sesame, pumpkin), whole grains, organ meats	Asthma, atherosclerosis, heart disease, headaches, insomnia, nervous & glandular disorders, poor circulation, premature aging, rheumatism, shortness of breath
C Ascorbic Acid Water Soluble	RDA SR 250–5,000 mg Toxicity	45 mg 5,000–15,000 mg	Citrus fruits, cantaloupe, green peppers, broccoli (cooked), papaya (raw), strawberries	Allergies, anemia, atherosclerosis, arthritis, baldness, bleeding gums, bruises, capillary wall ruptures, colds, cystitis, dental cavities, hypoglycemia, heart disease, hepatitis, low infection resistance, nosebleeds, poor digestion, obesity, prickly heat, sinusitis, tooth decay
D Fat Soluble	RDA SR Toxicity	400 IU 500–1,500 IU 2,500 IU	Egg yolks, organ meats, bone meal, sunlight, liver (beef), milk, salmon/tuna (canned)	Acne, allergies, arthritis, burning sensation (mouth & throat), cystitis, diarrhea, eczema, insomnia, myopia, nervousness, poor metabolism, psoriasis, softening bones & teeth

Vitamin	Daily Dosage	Sources	Deficiency Symptoms
E Tocopherol Fat Soluble	RDA 12–15 IU SR 50–600 IU Toxicity 4,000–30,000 IU	Dark green vegetables, eggs, liver, organ meats, wheatgerm, vegetable oils, dessicated liver, oatmeal (cooked), safflower oil, vegetable oils, peanut (roasted with skin), tomatoes, wheatgerm oil	Allergies, arthritis, atherosclerosis, baldness, cross eyes, cystitis, diabetes, dry, dull, or falling hair, enlarged prostate gland, gastrointestinal disease, heart disease (coronary, thrombosis, angine pectoris, rheumatic heart disease), impotency, menstrual problems, menopause, migraine headaches, miscarriages, muscular wasting sterility, myopia, obesity, phlebitis, sinusitis, stress, thrombosis, varicose veins, warts, wrinkles
F Unsaturated fatty acids Fat Soluble	RDA none stated SR 10% total calories Toxicity not known	Vegetable oils (safflower, soy, corn), wheat germ, sunflower seeds	Acne, allergies, baldness, bronchial asthma, diarrhea, dry skin, dry brittle hair, eczema, gall bladder problems, heart disease, leg ulcers, nail problems, psoriasis, rheumatoid arthritis, obesity, varicose veins, weight loss
K Menadione Fat Soluble	RDA none stated SR 300–500 mcg Toxicity not known	Green leafy vegetables, safflower oil, blackstrap molasses, yogurt, oatmeal, liver (beef)	Bruises, diarrhea, gall stones, increased tendency to hemmorrhage, menstrual problems, miscarriages, nosebleeds

Mineral	Daily Dosage	Sources	Deficiency Symptoms
Calcium	RDA 800–1,400 mg SR 1,000–2,000 mg Toxicity —	Milk, cheese, molasses, yogurt, bone meal, dolomite, almonds, American cheese, liver (beef)	Arthritis, aging symptoms (backache, bone pain, finger tremors), foot/leg cramps, heart palpitations, insomnia, menstrual cramps, menopause problems, muscle cramps, arm & leg numbness, nervousness, obesity, premenstrual tension, rheumatism, tooth decay
Chromium	RDA none stated SR 100–300 mcg Toxicity not known	Brewer's yeast, clams, corn oil, whole grain cereals	Atherosclerosis, glucose intolerance in diabetics, hypoglycemia
Copper	RDA 2 mg SR 2–4 mg Toxicity 40 mg	Legumes, nuts, organ meats, seafood, raisins, molasses, bone meal, Brazil nuts, soybeans	Anemia, baldness, impaired respiration, skin sores, weakness
Iodine	RDA 100–130 mcg SR 100–1,000 mcg Toxicity not known	Seafood, kelp tablets, salt (iodized)	Atherosclerosis, cold hands & feet, dry hair, goiter, hyperthyroidism, irritability, nervousness, obesity
Iron	RDA 10–18 mg SR 15 mg–50 mg Toxicity 100 mg	Blackstrap molasses, eggs, fish, organ meats, poultry, wheat germ, dessicated liver, shredded wheat	Anemia, breathing difficulties, brittle nails, colitis, iron deficiency anemia (pale skin, fatigue), constipation, menstrual problems

Mineral	Daily Dosage	Sources	Deficiency Symptoms
Magnesium	RDA 300–350 mg SR 300–350 mg Toxicity 30,000 mg	Bran, honey, green vegetables, nuts, seafood, spinach, bone meal, kelp tablets, bran flakes, peanuts (roasted with skin), tuna fish (canned)	Confusion, depression, disorientation, heart conditions, irritability, kidney stones, nervousness, prostate troubles, rapid pulse, sensitivity to noise, stomach acidity, tooth decay, obesity, tremors
Manganese	RDA none stated SR 1–50 mg Toxicity —	Bananas, bran, celery, cereals, egg yolks, green leafy vegetables, legumes, liver, nuts, pineapples, whole grains	Ataxia (muscle coordination failure), allergies, asthma, diabetes, dizziness, ear noises, fatigue, loss of hearing
Phosphorous	RDA 800 mg SR 800–1,000 mg Toxicity not known	Eggs, fish, grains, glandular meats, meat, poultry, yellow cheese, calf liver, milk/yogurt, eggs (cooked)	Appetite loss, arthritis, fatigue, irregular breathing, nervous disorders, obesity, stunted growth in children, stress, tooth & gum disorders, weight loss
Potassium	RDA none stated SR 100–300 mg Toxicity not known Average daily intake 1,950–5,850 mg	Dates, figs, peaches, tomato juice, blackstrap molasses, peanuts, raisins, seafood, apricots (dried), bananas, flounder (baked), potatoes (baked), sunflower seeds	Acne, allergies, burns, colic in infants, constipation, dry skin, diabetes, high blood pressure, heart disease (angine pectoris, congestive heart failure, myocardial infarction), general weakness, insomnia, muscle damage, nervousness, slow irregular heartbeat, thirst, weak reflexes

Mineral	Daily Dosage	Sources	Deficiency Symptoms
Sodium	RDA none stated SR 100–300 mg Toxicity 14,400 mg Average daily intake 2,800–6,900 mg	Salt, milk, cheese, seafood	Appetite loss, dehydration, fever, heat stroke, intestinal gas, muscle shrinkage, vomiting, weight loss
Sulphur	RDA none stated SR trace Toxicity not known	Bran, cheese, clams, eggs, nuts, fish, wheat germ	Arthritis, skin disorders (eczema, dermatitis, psoriasis)
Zinc	RDA 15 mg SR 20–100 mg Toxicity not known	Brewer's yeast, liver, seafood, soybeans, spinach, sunflower seeds, mushrooms	Atherosclerosis, baldness, cirrhosis, delayed sexual maturity, diabetes, fatigue, high cholesterol level, infertility, loss of taste, poor appetite, prolonged wound healing, retarded growth, sterility

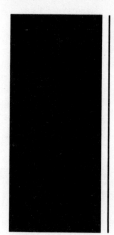

Index